"Metacognitive therapy (MCT) is based on a psychological model for how humans process information and specify how related psychological processes are affected across mental disorders. The clear scientific foundation, combined with related clinical interventions, is bringing the field of treating mental disorders forward. Göran Parment's years of clinical experience clearly shine through in his writing, making it an easy read with high relevance for clinical practice across a wide range of mental disorders and psychological problems."

Odin Hjemdal, *PhD, and specialist in clinical psychology, professor of clinical psychology at NTNU, Norwegian University of Science and Technology, Trondheim, Norway*

"Metacognitive therapy (MCT) is a research-oriented psychological treatment, developed from the bottom up based on key psychological processes. Göran Parment has extensive clinical experience, which is truly evident in this specific book. For clinicians who want to bridge the gap between research and clinical practice in MCT, this is the book to read."

Sverre Urnes Johnson, *PhD, professor of clinical psychology at the University of Oslo*

"Encompassing both theoretical model and concepts and clinical case examples, this is an excellent introduction to metacognitive therapy, indispensable for everyone interested in this innovative treatment approach—researchers, clinicians, and students alike. The author is especially commended for putting an emphasis on transdiagnostic perspectives."

Benjamin Bohman, *PhD, associate professor in clinical psychology at Karolinska Institutet, Stockholm, Sweden*

I0130604

Metacognitive Therapy

Metacognitive Therapy is an indispensable guide both for experienced and newly trained therapists who sometimes feel stuck or who are looking for a clear roadmap for conceptualizing and treating complex and comorbid problems.

Drawing on the transdiagnostic approach pioneered by Wells in 2009, Göran Parment uses his extensive clinical experience to guide the reader through the core concepts in MCT, illustrating the theoretical model with clinical examples and references to the latest evidence-based research. The book points out the significant transdiagnostic possibilities across disorders and shows how MCT can be applied to a wide array of common clinical disorders and comorbidities. The case formulation and the therapeutic procedures and applications are illustrated with clinical vignettes and therapist–client dialogues.

The book also discusses common doubts and questions about MCT's application as well as MCT's potential as a paradigm-shifting form of psychotherapy.

Göran Parment is an experienced licensed psychologist, a specialist in clinical psychology, and a MCTI-registered therapist at an advanced level. He is engaged as a lecturer and supervisor at the Metacognitive Therapy Institute.

Clinical Topics in Psychology and Psychiatry

Series Editor: Bret A. Moore, PsyD, Boulder Crest Retreat, Virginia, USA

Much of the available information relevant to mental health clinicians is buried in large and disjointed academic textbooks and expensive and obscure scientific journals. Consequently, it can be challenging for the clinician and student to access the most useful information related to practice. **Clinical Topics in Psychology and Psychiatry** includes authored and edited books that identify and distill the most relevant information for practitioners and presents the material in an easily accessible format that appeals to the psychology and psychiatry student, intern or resident, early career psychologist or psychiatrist, and the busy clinician.

Socratic Questioning for Therapists and Counselors
Learn How to Think and Intervene Like a Cognitive Behavior Therapist
Scott H. Waltman, R. Trent Codd, III, Lynn M. McFarr, and Bret A. Moore

Technology and Mental Health
A Clinician's Guide to Improving Outcomes
Edited by Greg M. Reger

Racism and African American Mental Health
Using Cognitive Behavior Therapy to Empower Healing
Janeé M. Steele

Metacognitive Therapy
Modern Approaches for Transdiagnostic Case Formulation and Treatment
Göran Parment

Practical Psychopharmacology, 2nd edition
Basic to Advanced Principles
Nevena V. Radonjić, Jeffrey S. MacDaniels, and Thomas L. Schwartz

For more information about this series, please visit: www.routledge.com/Clinical-Topics-in-Psychology-and-Psychiatry/book-series/TFSE00310

Metacognitive Therapy
Modern Approaches for Transdiagnostic Case Formulation and Treatment

Göran Parment

Routledge
Taylor & Francis Group

NEW YORK AND LONDON

Designed cover image: Getty Images

First published in English 2026
by Routledge
605 Third Avenue, New York, NY 10158

and by Routledge
4 Park Square, Milton Park, Abingdon, Oxon OX14 4RN

Routledge is an imprint of the Taylor & Francis Group, an informa business

© 2026 Göran Parment

Published in Swedish by Studentlitteratur AB [2023]

ISBN: 978-1-032-98114-7 (hbk)
ISBN: 978-1-032-98113-0 (pbk)
ISBN: 978-1-003-59710-0 (ebk)

DOI: 10.4324/9781003597100

Typeset in Sabon
by Taylor & Francis Books

Contents

Figures

Series Editor's foreword

Metacognitive Therapy: Modern Approaches for Transdiagnostic Case Formulation and Treatment is the latest volume in one of Routledge's most popular series, Clinical Topics in Psychology and Psychiatry (CTPP). The overarching goal of CTPP is to provide mental health practitioners with practical information on pharmacological and psychological topics. Each volume is comprehensive but easy to digest and integrate into day-to-day clinical practice. It is multidisciplinary, covering topics relevant to the fields of psychology and psychiatry, and appeals to the student, novice, and senior clinician. Books chosen for the series are authored or edited by national and international experts in their respective areas, and contributors are also highly respected clinicians. The current volume exemplifies the intent, scope, and aims of the CTPP series.

In the current volume, Swedish psychologist, educator, and clinical supervisor Göran Parment relies on his decades of experience in the areas of cognitive-behavioral therapy (CBT) and metacognitive therapy. The latter, developed in the 1990s by Adrian Wells, is a particular form of psychotherapy that teaches individuals how to modify metacognitive beliefs (i.e. what patients believe about their thoughts and their thinking process) to alleviate worry, anxiety, and other distressing symptoms. Aligned with CBT, metacognitive therapy differs from the former in that it is more of a process-oriented approach to understanding the role of thinking and psychological distress, whereas CBT is more content focused.

One of the features of this book that will be most rewarding is the richness of the experiences and understanding the author brings to the volume. Parment relies on his extensive work as a clinician and clearly illustrates the core tenets of metacognitive therapy through thoughtful and relevant clinical examples. However, he does not rely on clinical examples and anecdotal stories alone to make his points. The reader will realize early on that Parment is well versed in the research supporting the theory and practice of CBT in general and metacognitive therapy specifically. Upon finishing this book, the reader will come to understand that metacognitive therapy is evidence-based, practical and intuitive, transdiagnostic, and highly effective.

The reader will find that this volume flows seamlessly and helps the reader develop in their understanding of the material. This seamlessness is a result of the author's careful selection of chapter topics, methods of delivery and description, and his decades of experience. Parment speaks to you as a colleague, clinical supervisor, and educator. The chapters are written as if you were sitting across from him and enjoying an expert discussion about the material

I am convinced that *Metacognitive Therapy: Modern Approaches for Transdiagnostic Case Formulation and Treatment* will be one of the lead textbooks in this emerging area of clinical practice. It will also function as an excellent review for experienced practitioners looking for an easily digestible presentation of the latest science and thinking on the subject. Therapists already trained and practicing CBT will find this approach relatively easy to adapt into their current approach to working with clients from diverse backgrounds dealing with varied clinical concerns.

Bret A. Moore, PsyD, ABPP
Series Editor
Clinical Topics in Psychology and Psychiatry

Foreword

Göran Parment has the distinction of authoring the first Swedish book on Metacognitive Therapy (MCT). His work is a significant addition to the field, especially as a growing number of Swedish therapists have shown an increasing interest in MCT, incorporating it into their daily practice.

The availability of this resource in English is a commendable milestone. It's crucial to disseminate knowledge about MCT, given that research indicates its superior efficacy in treating anxiety disorders and depression compared to other methods. With over two decades of research in MCT, I can attest to its innovative approach in mental health treatment. MCT offers a fresh perspective, providing hope for many patients struggling with pervasive thoughts and distress characterized by worry, depressive rumination, and negative thinking patterns.

In this book, Göran Parment articulates the foundational tenets of Metacognitive Therapy (MCT) with many clinical examples that enrich therapeutic practice. He illustrates the potential of MCT in replacing outdated mental health management strategies with new, effective techniques that alleviate anxiety and depression. Central to MCT is the modulation of personal reactions to intrusive thoughts, anxiety, and discomfort, as these reactions determine the persistence or abatement of psychological issues. The book offers an accessible introduction to MCT's core concepts, distilling complex theories into clear, illustrative explanations. Drawing on the transdiagnostic approach pioneered by Wells in 2009, Parment demonstrates MCT's versatility in addressing a spectrum of disorders.

With his profound expertise in MCT, Parment describes its principles with precision. The book is replete with clinical vignettes and practical applications of MCT to common daily challenges, vividly brought to life through numerous therapist–client dialogues. His text aims to preserve the essence of the original content and shows how MCT can be applied across a wide range of conditions.

The book is suitable for readers such as psychology students and therapists because of its clinically oriented approach to the subject. Parment is a psychologist with extensive clinical experience, and he provides information from a broad spectrum of research within MCT. I recommend the book to anyone interested in MCT and I am sure that the reader will find good advice and examples that can be used both in private life and in clinical practice. MCT carries the important message that whether life is good or bad, people can learn to change their thinking patterns, which are at the core of mental health problems.

Hans M. Nordahl, Ph.D.
Professor, Norwegian University of Science and Technology

About the author

Göran Parment is an experienced licensed psychologist and psychotherapist, supervisor in CBT and MCT, specialist in clinical psychology and a MCTI® registered therapist at advanced level. He is engaged as a psychotherapy supervisor in different clinical settings, research projects, and psychology and psychotherapy programs. He is also engaged as a supervisor and teacher at the international MCT Institute. Göran is a board member of MCT-SE, the Swedish branch of the MCT Institute. He works in private practice in Stockholm, Sweden, and online, providing psychological treatment and supervision.

Introduction

The importance of metacognition in our lives

Metacognition matters. Metacognition can also be effectively altered, modified, in such a way that a spontaneous recovery from emotional problems and mental illness can take place. This is what this book is about, it's about metacognitive change. How the individual regulates his or her thought processes and attention, and how he or she relates to their thoughts and memories, is of crucial importance for the emotional well-being and otherwise functioning. Our way of relating to thoughts, impulses and memories affects the feeling of stress and our emotional experience of being secure or in danger. Metacognitive regulation has repercussions in family life, in the workplace and in studies. Perseverance, the ability to cope with adversity and to solve problems, is affected by metacognitive regulation. Our relationship with thoughts affects the perception we have of ourselves, the people around us, and how we take on the challenges and opportunities in our lives.

Why this book?

In 2023, when originally published (Parment, 2023), this was the first book on MCT written in Swedish. To my best knowledge, it even happened to be the first book worldwide in almost 15 years written and published for the clinical profession. That is, since the groundbreaking book *Metacognitive Therapy for Anxiety and Depression* by Adrian Wells (2009) and Fisher and Wells (2009). In this English translation, a few more recent references have been added. Also, some chapters have been broken up and shortened, and thus there are a few more chapters in this English edition. So far MCT has been disseminated the most in countries like Norway, Denmark and Germany. Today there is an increasing interest among psychology students, practicing psychologists and psychotherapists both in Sweden and in many other countries. MCT is furthermore increasingly in demand from clients and patient associations. Quite a few clinicians describe the encounter with MCT as a meeting with no return, i.e. many of them experience the model as providing them with a completely new and sharper understanding of

DOI: 10.4324/9781003597100-1

common clinical problems. MCT as a treatment model also has an interesting feature in its ability to attract psychologists and psychotherapists regardless of previous theoretical training. Among clinicians who have applied to, and graduated from the MCT training program, MCT Masterclass, many have done their original training and graduation in either cognitive behavioral therapy (CBT) or psychodynamic therapy (PDT). These clinicians have found that the MCT model provides better explanatory value, new tools in clinical situations, and that it is applicable across a wider range of psychological problems. MCT is effective. The benefits of transdiagnostic treatment are extensive.

A central reference in metacognitive therapy still is the book *Metacognitive Therapy for Anxiety and Depression*, published in 2009. It was written by the originator of MCT, Professor Adrian Wells. That book contains, in addition to a review of the theory, also protocols for the treatment of generalized anxiety disorder (GAD), post-traumatic stress disorder (PTSD), obsessive-compulsive disorder (OCD) and depression. For clinicians who want to learn and practice MCT, Wells (2009) is indispensable. Having said that the 2009 book is indispensable does not mean that it is sufficient. Psychologists and psychotherapists who want to acquire competence and skills to practice MCT, of course also need adequate training and supervision in the method. Formal training in MCT is only provided by the MCT Institute in Manchester and Trondheim. The title MCTI® Registered Therapist[1] shows that the clinician has attended and passed the MCT Masterclass. As a psychologist, giving the impression that you provide or conduct metacognitive therapy (MCT) and at the same time lacking adequate training and supervision in the method, can be considered contrary to professional ethical principles for psychologists, in the Nordic countries (Swedish Psychological Association, 1998) as well as in many other countries. See for example corresponding ethical guidelines by the American Psychological Association (2017), and the British Psychological Society (2021). These ethical guidelines set out, among other things, principles of professional competence, integrity, transparency and clarity regarding one's own qualifications.

Since Wells (2009), several important treatment studies have been published. Regarding the chosen research strategy for the development of MCT and the state of evidence in 2009, Wells wrote:

> There is currently a greater amount of data supporting the theory than there is data supporting the treatment. Moreover, the treatment data is based mainly on small experimental evaluations. This is an inevitable consequence of the systematic approach we have taken to treatment, development and evaluation.
>
> (Wells, 2009, p. 246)

As well as additional support for the theoretical model since 2009, several major treatment studies have now been published. In addition, Wells (2019) has updated and further refined the theoretical model on which MCT rests, the so-called S-REF model. The evidence for MCT as a treatment has strengthened significantly since 2009; see for example meta-analyses by Andersson et al. (2024) and Normann and Morina (2018). In several randomized and controlled studies, MCT has outperformed CBT in generalized anxiety disorder (GAD) (Af Winklerfelt Hammarberg et al., 2023; Nordahl, Borkovec et al., 2018; van der Heiden et al., 2012; Wells et al., 2010). MCT in social anxiety/social phobia has been proven more effective than drug treatment and the combination drug treatment + psychotherapy (Nordahl et al., 2016). In addition, studies have been published indicating that metacognitive change rather than cognitive change is the mediating factor in the treatment of social anxiety (Nordahl et al., 2017, 2022; Nordahl & Wells, 2017). MCT has also been compared with *prolonged exposure* (PE) in PTSD (Wells et al., 2015) and with *eye movement desensitization and reprocessing* (EMDR) (Nordahl, 2016), and in these studies MCT has been found superior to EMDR and at least equal compared to PE. MCT in depression appears to provide similar results (Jordan et al., 2014; Schaich et al., 2023) or better than CBT (Callesen et al., 2020a) and show more long-lasting treatment effects than other psychological treatments (Dammen et al., 2016; Solem et al., 2019). Anxiety and depression problems in patients with cardiovascular disease seem to be reduced more effectively with MCT than with other treatments (Wells et al., 2021). In a randomized controlled trial (Johnson et al., 2017), MCT as a transdiagnostic treatment has also been compared with specific evidence-based CBT protocols for panic disorder, PTSD and social phobia, and MCT was then found to be at least equally effective. Since 2009, very interesting treatment studies have also been published on MCT in OCD (Carter et al., 2022a; Exner et al., 2024; Glombiewski et al., 2021; Melchior et al., 2023; Papageorgiou et al., 2018; van der Heiden et al., 2016), substance abuse (Caselli et al., 2018) and personality syndromes (Nordahl et al., 2016; Nordahl & Wells, 2019).

There are very large patient populations that could be offered effective help with MCT. Although MCT has been found to be efficacious in disorders such as those just mentioned, it is misleading to limit the discussion on evidence to treatment of specific diagnoses. Metacognitive therapy is above all an evidence-based treatment to address transdiagnostic mechanistic processes beyond the diagnoses described in, for example, DSM 5 and ICD 10. In MCT, these transdiagnostic mechanistic processes are referred to as the CAS (the *cognitive attentional syndrome*) and dysfunctional metacognition. CAS is characterized by repetitive negative thinking in the form of worry and rumination which leads to attention being persistently locked to stimuli and themes that are perceived as threatening. According to MCT, CAS and dysfunctional metacognition are what cause and maintain emotional and psychological problems. CAS is driven by dysfunctional metacognition, by positive and negative metacognitive beliefs such as "By worrying, I am better prepared" or "I can't help but worry". Other metacognitive beliefs can be "Continued worry or rumination will ruin my health" or "Some thoughts are potentially dangerous to think". MCT is to be understood as an evidence-based treatment to reduce worry, rumination and other processes that are elements of the CAS. It is a model – the only one that exists and thus completely unique as a form of psychotherapy – designed to systematically modify dysfunctional metacognition. By reducing the CAS and dysfunctional metacognition, the causes of the symptoms and disorders are treated, and a natural recovery process can take place.

Bearing in mind that MCT and the S-REF model already from its original formulation – see for example Wells & Matthews (1994) – has been developed as a transdiagnostic model, this book further emphasizes and expands on the transdiagnostic perspective and the potential applications. A broad spectrum of common disorders and emotional problems is reviewed, discussed and illustrated through clinical vignettes and with many references to recent MCT research.

Intended audience

This book is aimed at both experienced psychologists, psychotherapists and other clinicians and those who are newly trained or in training. Hopefully, others who want to increase their understanding of MCT will also find it informative and useful.

Depending on the higher education context, the book can be included in curricula in psychology or psychotherapy courses as well as in coherent psychology programs. It can be used both as orientation and in-depth study. A book on MCT as a modern form of evidence-based psychological treatment should be of relevance to a large group of practicing clinicians. An increasing number of psychiatrists, psychologists and psychotherapists are turning their attention to MCT as a modern transdiagnostic treatment. Clients and patient associations are increasingly demanding MCT, and that is for very good reasons. MCT is an evidence-based and effective treatment that is widely applicable to many forms of psychological problems and to large patient groups.

MCT is of relevance, not least because the model is transdiagnostic, diagnosis-crossing. Transdiagnostic treatment is something very important considering that the most common situation in everyday clinical practice is comorbidity. More common than clients seeking help for only one psychological problem or disorder, is that they are bothered by several, for example both anxiety and depression, both obsessive thoughts and generalized anxiety, etcetera. If the therapist can help the client with several psychological problems at the same time, this is of course preferable. It also makes it easier for the clinician to achieve a high level of competence within one model instead of learning from many disorder-specific manuals. Unlike some current modular transdiagnostic treatment models, MCT is a theory-driven model. A thesis that will be pursued in this book is that a therapy model such as MCT, which is based on theory-driven empiricism, provides greater opportunities for development in the field of psychotherapy than eclectic technology- and module-based models.

The structure of the book

This book does not contain or reproduce already existing treatment protocols from Wells (2009). However, the clinical approach and the therapeutic techniques are described in detail. Since MCT is a theory-driven form of treatment where the interventions follow coherently from the theoretical model and case formulation, the treatment chapter is preceded by reviews of MCT as a theoretical model. Theoretical and methodological integrity are strongly emphasized in MCT. Treatment techniques from other psychotherapy models cannot be eclectically incorporated. The metacognitive dialogue is crucial in MCT. There are many clinical vignettes with fictitious dialogues between the client and therapist to make the theory and the therapeutic procedures more vivid for the reader. The book describes some further development and clarification of the theoretical model (Wells, 2019) since the groundbreaking book by Wells (2009). In addition, a further development of the treatment intervention *attention training technique* (ATT) is described. Although some further development and nuance has thus taken place, the model has been theoretically and methodologically stable over time. The central treatment interventions such as the metacognitive dialogue, *detached mindfulness* (DM) and various attentional techniques are delivered in principle in the same way today as in 2009.

Chapter 1 presents several vignettes in which various psychological problems of some fictional characters are described. Based on the usual DSM 5 or ICD 10 diagnostic systems, the problems could appear as quite different. The question gradually being raised is whether the problems really are diverse or whether there are instead common transdiagnostic processes beyond the DSM and ICD that, when made visible, will make the problems appear more similar than different. The chapter also contains arguments for transdiagnostic treatments, both in the sense of cross-diagnosis and in the sense of "processes beyond the DSM and ICD diagnoses".

Chapter 2 presents the theoretical model on which MCT is based, the S-REF model (*self-regulatory executive function model*; Wells & Matthews, 1994, 1996). This chapter provides a closer look at the central concept CAS (*cognitive attentional syndrome*) and how repetitive negative thinking such as worry, rumination and threat monitoring are assumed to explain a wide range of emotional and psychological problems. It also describes how CAS is to be understood as a voluntarily controlled and goal directed response to spontaneous negative thoughts, so-called trigger thoughts or negative automatic thoughts, such thoughts that we all experience daily and hence could be regarded as normal phenomena. In addition, the crucial importance of metacognition and how CAS is explained by metacognitive processes is described. As mentioned earlier, MCT is a theory driven model. Without a sound understanding and strong anchoring in the S-REF model, it is not possible to carry out MCT with the intended precision and quality.

Chapter 3 presents overall treatment objectives, principles and interventions, as well as the structure of the treatment course and of the treatment session. The case formulation in MCT and the socialization to the model is described. The therapeutic interventions in MCT are described and several vignettes are included to illustrate. The metacognitive dialogue is fundamental in MCT. That dialogue should be exploratory and designed to give the clients the opportunity to discover their relationship to thoughts and how the regulation of cognition affects emotional regulation and perception of the patient's own abilities. Furthermore, this dialogue is used to make it possible to discover that it is the relationship to thoughts and thinking that constitutes problems in our lives rather than the events we encounter or the cognitions per se. Various negative life events occur in the life of every human being of course, but worry, rumination, and other CAS reduce our ability to face and effectively deal with the challenges we meet. For most of us, it is unusual to reflect on how we relate to a negative thought. Even more so to converse with someone else about this. Through the metacognitive exploratory dialogue, the client is guided to discover and experiment with alternative approaches to thoughts and thinking, which will reduce the emotional problems, and which facilitate effective self-regulation and lead to a new and more helpful model of one's own mind.

Chapter 4 continues with presentations of therapeutic interventions and techniques. However, this chapter elaborates further on how the verbal and behavioral interventions in MCT are aimed at challenging and modifying dysfunctional metacognition. One of the most important interventions, Detached Mindfulness, is described, as well as interventions to increase flexibility and executive control of attention. This chapter ends with a paragraph on how therapeutic resistance and ambivalence towards change can be conceptualized and dealt with in MCT.

Chapter 5 presents how MCT can be used to conceptualize and treat various common anxiety and worry problems. In this chapter and the following Chapter 6, I want to guide the reader's attention to the many possibilities and rich potential of MCT. Chapters 5 and 6 point out the manifestations and expressions of the CAS and problematic metacognition in a wide range of clinical problems, starting with anxiety and worry problems in Chapter 5. MCT can be considered an evidence-based treatment to effectively reduce CAS and dysfunctional metacognition. Since CAS and dysfunctional metacognition appear to be significant processes in all clinical problems described in Chapters 5 and 6, the treatment implications and the new possibilities should be significant.

Chapter 6 continues from Chapter 5 with presentations on how MCT can be used for conceptualization and treatment, not only for anxiety and worry problems, but also for many other common clinical problems. This chapter presents applications of the S-REF model to disorders such as PTSD, OCD, depression, somatic health problems, personality disorders and more.

Chapter 7 presents the evidence for MCT, both the state of evidence for MCT as a theoretical model and for MCT as a psychological treatment. A strategy in the development of MCT has been for the model to be strongly theoretically grounded in experimental studies from cognitive psychology and from cognitive and metacognitive models of attention, thought processes and emotion. A vantage point has been that such an empirical theoretical approach should provide superior conditions for much-needed development in the field of psychotherapy. Many other psychotherapy models today lack this empirical theoretical basis and instead eclectically incorporate different therapeutic techniques that, to various degrees, have shown empirical support.

Chapter 8 gives examples of common initial misunderstandings regarding limitations of the applicability of MCT. Is MCT too difficult for many clients? Does the client need a very mature and sophisticated cognitive and metacognitive ability to respond to treatment? Conversely, it´s not uncommon to perceive MCT as a superficial and simplifying model that avoids the complexity of the human mind and experience. "But aren't emotional problems more than thoughts?" is one of the headings in this chapter.

In Chapter 9, MCT as an emerging new paradigm in the field of psychotherapy is further developed. This chapter provides a discussion on how MCT differs theoretically and practically from CBT and from the so-called "third wave CBT". The chapter ends with a look to future developments.

At the end of the book there are two appendices. Appendix 1 contains a list of the concepts in MCT and other abbreviations that occur. Appendix 2 describes instruments for measuring CAS and metacognition.

Thanks to

Having written this book, there are people that I´m deeply grateful to, starting with Professor Adrian Wells, who developed this highly effective form of psychological treatment. Listening to, discussing with and witnessing how Adrian describes and demonstrates MCT is always very engaging, informative and interesting. I would also like to thank Professor Hans M Nordahl, who was the one who directed my attention to MCT more than 10 years ago. Hans has given me very valuable supervision over the years. He has also been helpful with fact-checking of the original manuscript in Swedish and has provided valuable feedback to it. Other people I want to thank are my wife and MCT colleague Gunvor Mjös Parment. We have participated in MCT training together, we work together at our clinic with MCT and have had countless theoretical and clinical discussions to increase our understanding and competence. Gunvor has read and given useful comments on the text. Another very important colleague is Peter Myhr. Peter and I have also had countless conversations about MCT, we have, together with Gunvor, had collegial supervision and Peter and I have also jointly conducted many workshops on MCT in Sweden for psychologists in their clinical specialist training. Many of the ideas presented in the book are results of the discussions that Peter, myself and Gunvor have had together when exchanging experiences with each other. Peter has also been helpful in reading and giving valuable feedback on the book's manuscript. Thanks also to Ph.D. Bengt Eriksson who, maybe from more of an external perspective, has given very valuable feedback. Bengt has written books on psychotherapy models, their theoretical foundations and clinical applications, on eating disorders and on conceptualization in PDT and CBT. Bengt's areas of interest include schema therapy and integrative therapy. Another MCT colleague who has read and given valuable comments is Erling Hansen. This has been a process in which the text has been edited several times and where colleagues have left comments at different stages of the writing. There are probably still parts that could have been presented differently, more clearcut, or more elegant. For the less fortunate parts of the text that may still exist, I take sole responsibility.

Note

1 A list of registered MCT therapists in different countries can be found at www.mct-institute.co.uk.

1 The field of psychotherapy
From disparate problems to a unifying approach

Many and disparate problems or just a few similar ones?

In the psychiatric diagnostic systems DSM 5 and ICD 10, there are categories such as specific phobias, panic disorder with and without agoraphobia, post-traumatic stress disorder (PTSD), obsessive-compulsive disorder (OCD), social phobia/social anxiety, generalized anxiety disorder (GAD) and major depression. Approximately 25–30 percent of those who contact a health center in Sweden have been estimated in various studies to suffer from a mental illness (Socialstyrelsen, 2019). If you seek help for mental illness in primary care, antidepressants and/or various forms of psychological treatment are often prescribed. Psychological treatment such as CBT can often be offered in the form of treatment protocols aimed at specific psychiatric diagnoses. It's not unusual that various forms of brief or simplified psychological interventions are offered in primary care (at least in Scandinavia). These interventions are often based on a weak or even unknown state of evidence.

There are several evidence-based treatments for specific disorders such as panic disorder, social anxiety, obsessive-compulsive disorder, major depression, etcetera. However, among most clients seeking help for impaired mental health, the difficulties are not limited to just one mental health problem or specific disorder. Instead, what is more common is comorbidity, which means that one disorder usually coexists with at least one other disorder. For example, people who suffer from depressive disorders very often also experience various forms of anxiety problems. Furthermore it's common for mental health problems to coexist with somatic conditions or substance abuse/addiction. The phenomenon of comorbidity does not always need to be understood as an increase in the clients' total burden of problems. Instead, there is an ongoing debate in clinical psychology and in psychiatry about the fact that the current diagnostic systems are plagued with a lot of imperfections and that the divisions between different forms of psychiatric disorder often seem to be artificial and arbitrary.

Criticism of the current diagnostic system does not stop at a debate but has also developed into new research fields such as RDoC, *research domain criteria*, on genetic, neuropsychological factors and self-reported data behind

DOI: 10.4324/9781003597100-2

psychiatric problems. Another new field of research and a new diagnostic system based on the problems with DSM and ICD is HiTOP, *hierarchical taxonomy of psychopathology*; see for example Conway et al. (2019, 2022). However, HiTOP still appears to be a mainly unexplored diagnostic system in relation to the field of psychotherapy.

Metacognitive therapy (MCT) is a transdiagnostic treatment for various forms of emotional problems, impaired mental health and psychiatric disorders. Treatment studies of MCT have so far been conducted mostly for various types of anxiety problems and depression. In the case of generalized anxiety disorder GAD, which is characterized by persistent anxiety and difficult-to-control worry, the evidence supporting MCT can now be considered as strong. In several head-to-head clinical trials by independent research groups, the treatment has outperformed CBT (Af Winklerfelt Hammarberg et al., 2023; Nordahl, Borkovec et al., 2018; van der Heiden et al., 2012; Wells et al., 2010).

MCT as "transdiagnostic" means that the treatment targets comorbidity. The transdiagnostic perspective can also be understood as assessment and treatment being directed towards processes beyond the different symptoms described in the DSM and ICD systems. The cross-diagnosis, "beyond-processes" that are identified and treated in MCT are those described in the so-called S-REF model, the theoretical model on which MCT is based. The S-REF model will be explained in detail in Chapter 2. The treatment principles of MCT can most often be applied regardless of psychiatric diagnosis and even if the client meets diagnostic criteria for several disorders, i.e. even if the problems are comorbid. MCT can also be applied beyond psychiatric diagnoses, for example in cases where problems are experienced such as negative self-image, relationship difficulties, etcetera.

Below, some vignettes will be presented where we get to know Bengt, Aysha, Jessica and several other of our fellow human beings. All vignettes are fictitious, but if there are still recognition effects, it is probably because we humans are related in our emotional dispositions and in our predicaments. A premise in MCT is that the differences between diverse forms of mental health problems are less important than the similarities. Are there many different clinical difficulties that are portrayed in the vignettes that follow or is it possible to see a set of unifying mechanisms and to formulate them as just a few common problems? That is a question that we will come back to.

Bengt, 45, generally feels low and gloomy. Was this how he had imagined his life to be? What is it all about? Work, keep track of the teenage sons who don't really take care of their school duties. Pay the bills and then get old and die? What is the point with everything? Sure, you can meet up with old friends sometimes, have a drink or two with them, but everything feels more and more empty, like temporary diversions and distractions. He often stays in bed and dwells on themes like these in the mornings when he wakes up too early and feels creeping anxiety. Bengt suspects that he has inherited his mother's tendency to depression. His mother used to be emotionally absent during her episodes of depression.

Aysha almost always feels anxious, tense and insecure. It's as if she's constantly prepared to receive news of a deatht or a message that someone in the family is in serious trouble. She suffers from pain and a poor appetite. Aysha sleeps poorly and usually feels tired and exhausted. She feels guilty and shameful when she believes that she spreads more negative than positive energy to the rest of the family. Aysha takes some medications for her anxiety and depression, but she is not sure if they help. She seems to understand where the fears and pessimism come from. Her upbringing was anything but safe and stable.

Jessica finds it almost impossible to find stable and safe love relationships. It's as if she knows that she will always be alone and whatever intimate relationship she tries to build is doomed to fail. As if it's only a matter of time before her partner will get tired of her and leave her. She knows she is too much with all her emotions, and it can often lead to grueling scenes and difficult fights. Jessica spends a lot of time thinking about what true intentions her partner might have and whether they are honest in what they say to her. She is extremely vigilant about the tone of voice, glances and pauses that arise in conversations. She often thinks "it's really just as well to break up now at once instead of getting devastated later". She also becomes preoccupied with the thought that she will appear ridiculous and pitiful if she is left by a partner whom she has fallen in love with.

Fernando basically likes his work. If it weren't for the coffee breaks when you are supposed to be social and chat with colleagues. And if it weren't for the Thursday meetings, when you are expected to show the rest of the team how far you have come with your project. Ideally, you should sound enthusiastic and relaxed during your presentation, at least if you go by how others seem to behave in these situations. Fernando endures such meetings but finds them very stressful and demanding. He feels stuck, tense and ridiculously nervous. Sometimes, both on Friday and over the rest of the weekend, he feels ruined when he dwells on how nervously and strangely he conducted his presentation. Fernando's sister, who works in healthcare, has discussed with him whether he might suffer from some form of high-functioning autism. She points out that he never really seems to have appreciated social interaction to any great extent.

Ulla no longer recognizes herself. She has always been a high achiever, something of a mentor to her colleagues and the one who took the main responsibility and organized life in her family. She believes that she suffers from brain stress. She doesn't feel alert anymore after resting, finds it impossible to concentrate, and she is bothered by the stress symptoms after the slightest effort or commitment. She is convinced that she still suffers because she didn't care to listen to her body's signals in time. She has been on sick leave after what she experienced as a collapse six months ago. On that occasion she found herself with the car keys in her hand one morning, not knowing where she was going. The whole thing was very scary, like a rug being pulled away from under her. This would have been a normal working day after several weeks of increased workload. In addition, her mother had passed away earlier in the year. Ulla worries a lot whether she will ever get well again.

Bob suffers from psychosis. He is very anxious and from time to time quite sure that other people on the bus and in the shopping center can hear his thoughts. It all becomes extremely uncomfortable, and he tries to keep track of his thoughts and to control and foresee them. He is convinced that others are mocking him for his thoughts and that they are planning different ways to continue to harass and ridicule him. Bob pays a lot of attention to how other people in his environment appear, where they direct their gaze and how they adjust their facial expressions when approaching and passing him. Bob can think about such things for hours and then he gets completely restless.

What is similar and what is different in the vignettes? At first glance and based on the common diagnostic systems of DSM and ICD, they seem to illustrate several different problems. But are the difficulties fundamentally different? How could one conceptualize the origin of the problems and the reasons that they get persistent instead of temporary? To what degrees do biological and genetic factors contribute? Which of the problems are due to stressful and current negative life events? Which of the problems are caused by adverse childhood experiences? Which ones are most likely linked to social difficulties? For those who seek professional help with several concurrent problems as above, it is most often difficult to determine: What was the cause of the problems and what can be done to alleviate them? Which problems are the original or the most important and which can be understood as secondary and hence dependent on the primary ones? Is it possible to get help with several problems at the same time?

Both the client and the therapist will have pre-understandings of what constitutes, causes and perpetuates psychological problems. These preunderstandings may have been elaborated and reflected on to various degrees. Also, about treatment, the patient and the therapist will have various pre-understandings. How the problems are defined and conceptualized is of crucial importance when it comes to the possibilities of offering effective treatment. In the following vignette, psychologist Maja experiences several troublesome dilemmas in her professional practice.

Maja is a psychologist in a mental health clinic and has been trained in CBT. In the clinic, she meets clients who may have similar problems to those described in the previous vignettes. Of course, she also meets clients with several other problems. Some of her clients have problems with alcohol, are depressed, suffer relationship problems and are also bothered by anxiety, stress and worry. All these problems occur simultaneously and sometimes even a few more occur, such as sleep problems and fatigue. Maja is supposed to adhere to evidence-based clinical practice and to various CBT protocols. Despite her previous education and extensive training, she often finds her clinical tasks very demanding. A significant challenge is that the clients' problems usually tend to be comorbid. It is very rare that she meets clients who are bothered by only one specific disorder, such as social phobia. Although she is familiar with several evidence-based treatment protocols, she feels that it can be arbitrary how she then chooses between them or between different therapeutic techniques. Often, she finds herself using only certain techniques from different protocols and sometimes she integrates selected techniques from different treatment protocols, and that is because she rarely feels that the clients' problems completely fit the target group for a particular evidence-based protocol. She understands that eclectically incorporating techniques from different protocols can be a departure from an evidence-based approach, but what else could she do? She does not feel that her considerations in these clinical choice situations follow systematic and scientifically based principles. Hopefully, she has acquired good judgement after her long clinical training, but how can she know if her own judgment is superior or equal to that of a colleague who handles corresponding clinical choices in different ways? If a client were to suffer from both social phobia and obsessive-compulsive disorder, she would not be sure what problem she should try to treat first. In such a situation, she would also be uncertain whether she is expected to carry out two different treatments, one for social phobia and one for obsessive-compulsive disorder. If so, which of the treatments should she begin with? In addition, if the client has sleep problems, can she add a concomitant evidence-based treatment for sleep problems?

Transdiagnostic perspectives on problems and treatment

Psychologist Maja's various dilemmas in the previous vignette clarify some of the problems with diagnosis-specific treatments based on the DSM or ICD systems. The DSM and ICD systems can be understood as medical/psychiatric categorization models, but they do not explain the psychological mechanisms behind one or several diagnoses that are in focus. Applied in the field of psychological treatment, these diagnostic systems cannot provide an in-depth understanding of problematic psychological processes, nor a more precise guide to appropriate and targeted treatment interventions. The DSM system has enabled the field of psychotherapy to develop in such ways that it made it possible to compare the effects of psychotherapy at the group level with pharmacological treatment. For example, the work of Aaron Beck and colleagues was very important when they were able to demonstrate that CBT gave equivalent or better results than drugs for patients with a depression diagnosis according to the DSM (Beck et al., 1979). Authors such as Bakker (2019, 2022) also argue for the need for psychological explanatory models, rooted in clinical psychology, instead of medical ones, in order to enable continued theoretical-clinical development in the field of psychotherapy.

In addition to the problems already mentioned with DSM and ICD diagnostics, diagnosis-specific treatment protocols do not provide guidance on how comorbidities can be managed. In recent years, different transdiagnostic perspectives on treatment have emerged (see e.g. Dalgleish et al., 2020; Sauer-Zavala et al., 2017). Several arguments for the development of transdiagnostic perspectives have been put forward. One argument is that the diagnostic categories according to the DSM and ICD have indeed increased the reliability between assessors and clinicians, but that this has been at the expense of external validity and generalizability; That is, the problems that clients seek help for in everyday clinical practice are rarely clearly limited to just one diagnosis. The diagnostic categories could rather be seen as trivial variations and expressions of more underlying transdiagnostic syndromes and processes. When comorbidity seems to be the rule rather than the exception, this suggests that the existence of concomitantly delimited diagnoses is more to be understood as an artefact, derived from the design of diagnostic systems, than as an expression of the co-occurrence of genuinely delimited syndromes.

Furthermore, it is pointed out that the diagnoses are very heterogeneous. The diagnoses are made based on several criteria that must be met. They say nothing about the etiology, about the causes of the problems, and thus do not give any guidance on how the problems should be treated. How can you treat effectively if you do not know the causes of the psychological problem? For example, in the case of the diagnosis of major depressive disorder, it is found that two individuals who both meet the diagnostic criteria can potentially have only one symptom out of nine possible in common. When it comes to the diagnosis of borderline personality disorder according to DSM 5, five out of nine diagnostic criteria must be met. This means that there are 256 possible combinations of diagnostic criteria, all of which imply a fulfilled diagnosis. Dalgleish et al. (2020) point out that the function of any diagnostic system should be to increase the understanding of a complex problem, but that this heterogeneity within the diagnostic categories entails strong doubts about the usefulness of the DSM and ICD diagnoses.

In addition to the problems raised in the previous paragraphs, which present significant challenges for clinicians trained in diagnosis-specific treatment protocols, there are also other arguments for transdiagnostic perspectives on psychotherapy. An ever-increasing number of evidence-based, diagnosis-specific treatments are being developed, but instead of this becoming an asset for clients and therapists, it can be perceived as a problem. In practice, it will be impossible for the individual clinician to achieve a high level of competence other than in a very limited number of these treatments. If transdiagnostic, broadly applicable treatment models can be shown to be effective, which seems to be the case (see e.g. Pearl & Norton, 2017), it will be significantly less resource-intensive to train psychologists and psychotherapists. A trained clinician should thus be able to treat more conditions and more clients with varied problems. Another argument is that if transdiagnostic perspectives can provide a better understanding of underlying common processes, this should enable shorter and more effective treatments. A further argument is that more developed transdiagnostic perspectives could reduce the gaps between research and clinic, i.e. facilitate the implementation of evidence-based treatments in everyday clinical practice. This argument is then based on the assumption that the problems with external validity and generalizability would be reduced with transdiagnostic treatment.

In the clarification of transdiagnostic processes in psychotherapy, some authors highlight the importance of distinguishing between descriptive and mechanistic transdiagnostic processes (for an overview, see e.g. Dalgleish et al., 2020). An analogy with a hypothetical plane crash is referred to here to clarify. Both engine failure and gravity can constitute causal explanations for a flight failure, but to increase future flight safety, the most appropriate thing will be to analyze how exactly the engine failure occurred and what can be done to prevent similar failures in the future. Mechanistic transdiagnostic processes in psychotherapy are those that are both causal in terms of mental health/illness and therapeutically meaningful to identify and try to influence.

Nolen-Hoeksema and Watkins (2011) argue that transdiagnostic processes can also be divided into distal and proximal respectively. Distal processes are those that can be considered to exist earlier in a causal chain leading to psychological problems, such as environmental risk factors during childhood or biological risk factors. Proximal processes are those that are closer in time and with fewer prior causal mechanisms, that is, more directly causing the psychological problems. Distal factors lead to psychological problems only via mediating proximal risk factors, while proximal risk factors directly cause psychopathology. Distal factors are usually independent of the individual's own actions, they rather happen to the individual. Proximal factors are variables within the individual, often influencing psychotherapy in a way that distal factors are not once they have occurred. Proximal factors that may be relevant in psychotherapy may include dysfunctional behaviors or bias in information processing or attention.

Some common transdiagnostic explanations for mental illness

Considering the problems of Bengt, Aysha, Jessica and the others in the opening vignettes, factors such as a history of past or more recent negative life events, socio-economic stressors and biological vulnerability often recur as plausible transdiagnostic explanations.

Social factors, and exposure to negative life events

We all face adversity in our lives. Hopefully, we will also experience love and caring and take part in events that are wonderful, fun, exciting and stimulating. Of course, you want more of the good moments, and it often feels like something positive per se to have opportunities to long for and coming events ahead, to look forward to. We feel good when being cared for and loved, when we can influence others and our environment, when we are able to reach out and help, and experience a sense of belonging to meaningful social contexts, when we are feeling competent and so on. At the same time, we know that it is not possible to live a life without setbacks, disappointments, different kinds of loss and other difficult events. There are many aspects of our lives that are difficult or even impossible for us to alter or influence. Some of us get more than our fair share of painful experiences, abuse, and unhappiness. Social vulnerability and social injustice, poverty, undignified working conditions, health problems and failing bodily functions, forced loneliness and poor interpersonal relationships constitute obvious strains. Perhaps the hardest of all is to be or to feel excluded from significant others and from belonging to a social group. It is well documented that there is generally a connection between negative life events, such as having been exposed to abuse and neglect while growing up, and mental illness. It is also well documented that many people who have been through difficult life events can still testify to mental well-being (see, for example, Galatzer-Levy et al., 2018). Some may even say that they have been strengthened in the face of adversity and that they have learned to appreciate life and can value life in new ways.

Genes, biology and brain chemistry

We all live with different genetic and biological constitutions. Of course, there are conditions like dementia, head trauma and other events that can objectively damage the brain structure, limit us and cause obvious disabilities. However, such factors are not enough to explain the difference between mental health and emotional problems in general. Although our biology naturally plays a role, there are extremely few forms of mental illness where only biological factors are considered decisive. For example, the so-called serotonin hypothesis, a hypothesis that depression is caused by too low levels of the neurotransmitter serotonin in the brain's synapses, has been widely questioned (see e.g. Cowen & Browning, 2015; Healy, 2015). In a systematic review of the support for the serotonin hypothesis, Moncrieff et al. (2022) concluded:

> The main areas of serotonin research provide no consistent evidence of there being an association between serotonin and depression, and no support for the hypothesis that depression is caused by lowered serotonin activity or concentrations.

The term "neuropsychiatric disorders" gives a strong indication that a biological causal relationship has been established for certain problems. Of course, the brain is involved in all sensory, motor, emotional and cognitive activity, both in cases of positive approaching behaviors and negative avoiding behaviors. Still, in the case of emotional problems, they usually are not labeled as "neuropsychiatric". The fact that the brain is involved in all behaviors and in all psychological events does not mean that such biological causal relationships have been established behind the disorders that are described as "neuropsychiatric". Neuropsychiatric diagnoses are made through behavioral observations, i.e. through anamnesis of behavior, psychological tests and clinical interviews. For most patients for whom neuropsychiatric diagnoses have been made, there are no direct observations that provide evidence that neurological dysfunction is causing the problems.

In addition to social and psychological factors, it is now well known that there are complex and interrelated relationships between genes and the environment. For example, epigenetics is a relatively new area of research that studies how genetic expressions can be altered by and interact with environmental factors. Rather than dwelling on the old classic question of whether mental illness is explained by nature or nurture, we are now exploring many interacting factors and multifactorial relationships. The modern view is that multi-factorial and mutual relationships lie behind the development and maintenance of mental illness and emotional problems. What happens to us affects our sensorimotor system and biochemical processes in the brain, which in turn affect our cognition and behavior, which then affect our environment and what then will happen to us again. Biochemical processes in the brain and the rest of the body affect emotion and behavior while we again affect our brain functions through behaviors and thinking. For example, we will change the processes in the brain if we drink alcohol, use narcotics or get insufficient nutrition. If we turn and keep our attention to potential threats in our environment, the processes in the brain and in our bodies will also change. When we interrupt repetitive negative thinking, rumination and worry, and instead pay attention to events outside ourselves, this is reflected in measurably altered brain activity (Knowles & Wells, 2018).

From historical, social and biological explanations to psychological ones

When searching for transdiagnostic mechanisms behind the problems of Bengt, Aysha, Jessica and the others in the previous vignettes, one can also look for psychological explanations. Historical, social or biological models are far from sufficient to explain mental illness, of course even less sufficient in providing precise guidance on what needs to be done in psychotherapy. As mentioned earlier, there are people who testify that the difficulties they have gone through have given them robustness, perseverance and a deepened ability to appreciate life's joys and beauty. In a psychotherapy context, it would neither be helpful nor make much sense to guide treatment planning either based on mechanisms such as negative life events or biological factors. From the distinction between descriptive and mechanistic transdiagnostic processes, it is safe to conclude that historical life events and biological conditions cannot be directly influenced in psychotherapy. They are to be seen as distal factors. However, those seeking psychological treatment usually have cognitions and ideas about how historical, social and biological factors have been significant, and still are, and how these have affected or limited their own opportunities in life.

Rather than one's biological constitution, social situation or history of negative life events per se, one can argue that it is how one views all this that affects mental well-being. In the literature on cognitive therapy, for example, a quote by the Stoic philosopher Epictetus (probably 55–135 A.D.) is often referred to: "It is not what happens to you, but how you react to it that matters." From an evolutionary point of view, humans should be expected to be well equipped to deal with external stressors. Historically, human beings, like other organisms, have been shaped and developed in environments that have been anything but pleasant and peaceful. Stone Age, Bronze Age or 18th century humans should have faced significantly more external stressors in life than those people of today who live in economically well-developed social contexts and countries. Of course, variation exists, not all individuals will react in the same ways in face of negative life events. Not everyone will develop clinical depression after a relationship breakup or after becoming unemployed. Only a small percentage of those who have experienced a traumatic event seem to develop PTSD or other psychiatric problems (Breslau, 2002; Lassemo et al., 2017). In cognitive therapy and CBT, the focus is on how the individual thinks about different life events, about themselves and their own opportunities. Techniques that fall under the term "cognitive restructuring" are used in CBT to help the client reality test their cognitions and to think in a more balanced way about themselves, their history and others to alleviate psychological problems.

Cognitive and metacognitive processes

But is it really negative thoughts or is it rather problematic thinking that explains individual differences regarding vulnerability or resilience to mental illness? To clarify: We humans may have thoughts about, for example, being socially incompetent, sometimes based on negative life experiences. These, and related "I-am-incompetent" thoughts could be challenged in CBT by examining evidence for them reflecting truth or not, i.e. through techniques commonly referred to as cognitive restructuring. With this type of technique, the CBT therapist usually asks about experiences in the client's life that constitute evidence that the person is socially incompetent, as well as contradicting evidence that could lead to alternative thoughts and beliefs. However, if one lifts the gaze from the content of negative thoughts to a cognitive process level, it's also possible to examine negative thought processes on the theme of social incompetence. We can spend a lot of time worrying about our own social deficiencies and about how we may be perceived in certain social contexts. We can also continue thinking by analyzing the reasons for how we became incompetent. In metacognitive therapy, the focus is on negative thought processes instead of the content of negative thoughts. Based on metacognitive processes, we can also have different beliefs about the importance of negative thoughts, i.e. as very significant or instead as fundamentally trivial, possible to live with and possible to just notice and do nothing with.

Obviously, the individual's way of processing information will most significantly contribute to his or her emotional well-being. A person may hold very strong and definite ideas about the impact of negative childhood experiences and life events, or about imbalances in one's own biology or about dysfunctional brain activity, especially during periods of emotional suffering. For example, it is not uncommon for people who are bothered by psychological disorders to believe that something has gone wrong with their brains, that it has been damaged by stress, that serotonin levels are too low or that genes passed down from the parents' generation control their current mental health. Unfortunately, similar beliefs or hypotheses can also often be conveyed, almost as facts, via health care professionals, for example: "Your ADHD means that you have a limited attention span and a reduced capacity to stick to demanding tasks", "Your brain has become overloaded with too much stress. Now it is exhausted and needs a long recovery and rest from all stressors". Different conceptions of the self as damaged by difficult life events or by biological processes, could be described as cognitions within CBT. One could also look at the metacognitive processes and at the cognitions about one's own "mental apparatus", such as: "Because of what has happened to me/my damaged brain, I cannot regulate my attention, cannot stop worrying or ruminating, cannot choose to engage in my daily life instead", or "As long as I have thoughts about myself as socially defective, I can't function in normal social situations".

Regardless of the veracity of beliefs about a disturbed brain function, or a damaged brain, it's obvious that we are biological beings with the capacity to hold ideas about the same biology. Whether our brain is damaged by stress or not, whether our neurotransmitters are out of balance or not, we also have thoughts about how our brain and our biological processes work and affect our well-being. Based on this, we will have beliefs about our ability to influence and regulate our attention, our cognitive processes and our emotional well-being. We relate in different ways to various beliefs about our brain as healthy or damaged, or about our neurotransmitters as well-balanced or unbalanced. Thoughts that our biology or historical events control our emotional well-being are often difficult to perceive as ... well, thoughts. The capacity to pay attention for longer periods will of course vary based partly on biological factors and psychological maturity. But in addition, the individual has metacognitions about this cognitive ability, thoughts that one can relate to in different ways. For example, a person who experiences problems with concentration could interrupt his/her work during a difficult and challenging task when having thoughts such as "It's my ADHD, I just can't stick to the task and pay attention anymore" or "I just can't manage to be persistent in the work on a complicated and tedious task". In metacognitive therapy, one would explore whether it is possible not to respond to similar thoughts, i.e. relate to them as if they were not particularly important.

Declarative and procedural cognition and metacognition

In cognitive psychology, concepts such as declarative knowledge and procedural knowledge as well as explicit and implicit memories and beliefs are used. Declarative knowledge and explicit memories are those we are clearly aware of and that we can articulate in words. Procedural knowledge, on the other hand, is practical knowledge, knowledge of execution, and it is not primarily verbally formulated. A good craftsman, musician or athlete usually does not find it easy to formulate his or her full knowledge in words. It is not possible to explain exactly what you do when riding a bicycle and keeping your balance during the ride. That is, it becomes meaningful to talk about knowledge even when it becomes difficult or impossible to fully formulate in words. Like procedural knowledge, implicit memories are those that can be demonstrated without being consciously and verbally formulated. In cognitive psychology, it has also been possible to demonstrate that the concept of implicit memories and beliefs becomes useful and meaningful, possible to do research on and study the effects of; see for example Schacter et al. (1993). This book is about the importance of metacognition for psychological regulation. Many of the metacognitive regulatory processes are procedural. In MCT, metacognitive processes are examined, and in the therapeutic dialogue, one goal is to increase metacognitive awareness, i.e. towards raising procedural processes to the declaratory level. After explorations and modifications within the declarative knowledge system, the altered metacognitive processes are assumed to return to the predominantly procedural level. A person who, after successful MCT has reduced worry and rumination and who has discovered that negative thoughts can be safely left alone without further processing, is developing new ways of relating to thoughts, ways that over time will be experienced as safe and less tiresome, new habits that are most often unnecessary to reflect much on at a declarative level of knowledge.

2 Metacognitive therapy

A theory-driven transdiagnostic model

The fact that the model is theory-driven and generated from research-based information processing theories makes it fundamentally different from other existing psychotherapy models. One can assume that the conditions for real development in the psychotherapy field will improve considerably with this foundation in experimental studies and research-based theory. The fact that such a development is required is pointed out by, among others, Holmes et al. (2018), who note that although evidence-based treatments have been developed, the effect of these is far from satisfactory. In addition, Holmes and others highlight the importance of experimentally based theory development in the field of psychotherapy. If it is possible to gain a more precise, empirically grounded understanding of the mechanisms behind psychological problems, therapeutic interventions can be targeted directly and systematically towards changing them. Many contemporary evidence-based psychotherapy models are instead eclectic and technology- or modular-based. That is, they are centered around several techniques or modules that, based on observational studies, have been shown to work for many individuals, even if the mechanisms of change are unknown and theoretically unclear.

MCT has been developed methodically from the basis where theoretical concepts and mechanisms have been evaluated experimentally and step-by-step. The therapeutic techniques have been studied from smaller case series studies to larger controlled studies, which have enabled a systematic and research-based theory development (see, for example, Capobianco & Nordahl, 2023; Wells, 2019).

Other psychotherapy models in the 1990s often described problems with attention bias in terms of "bottom-up models", that is, as the result of reflexive processes stemming from emotion, personality, or environmental factors. The theoretical model for MCT, the S-REF model, is instead a "top-down model" that is based on the research-based knowledge of attentional and thought processes as largely voluntary. It is a model that describes in detail an architecture with different levels of cognition, how cognitive processes are controlled and regulated, and how attention bias and negative thought processes can cause emotional and psychological problems.

DOI: 10.4324/9781003597100-3

The transdiagnostic processes identified in MCT are partly those that are included in the concept of CAS (*cognitive attentional syndrome*) and partly dysfunctional metacognitive processes that are assumed to control CAS. CAS is to be understood as maladaptive self-regulation that results in emotional and psychological problems. The cognitive attentional syndrome CAS is characterized by repetitive negative thinking, especially worry and rumination. CAS is also characterized by the attention being persistently locked to what is perceived as threat and danger. Attentional resources are used in a threat-monitoring way and, during CAS activation, also tends to be internally directed towards thoughts, feelings and body sensations. Hence, threat monitoring can be directed to both external and internal perceived threats. From this follows that CAS apparently is not a balanced thinking style, but instead biased to potential threats. The concept of CAS also includes unhelpful thought control strategies such as thought suppression, excessive reasoning and counterproductive behaviors, such as alcohol use, excessive reassurance seeking, or avoidance. Similar strategies are used to deal with negative thoughts and to regulate negative thought processes. CAS is a toxic thinking style. It is assumed to constitute the difference between psychological well-being and emotional problems/psychological disorder. Most people can of course recognize themselves as occasional worriers or ruminators, but in mental illness these thought processes become perseverative and are used in much more inflexible ways.

So, if tiresome and even toxic, then why does the individual engage in the Cognitive Attentional Syndrome? In MCT, CAS is explained by meta-cognitive processes. Metacognition can be understood as cognition applied to cognition, as thinking about thinking or as regulating thinking with cognition. According to the theoretical model of MCT, CAS is controlled and regulated by metacognition, by positive and negative metacognitive beliefs. Examples of positive metacognitive beliefs can be: "By worrying, I am better prepared when problems arise" or "If I continue to analyze why I feel depressed, I will find answers that will help me get out of depression". Two types of negative metacognitive beliefs are described in the theoretical model: Meta-beliefs about CAS as uncontrollable, and beliefs about CAS as dangerous and harmful. An example of an uncontrollability meta-belief can be: "My worry just comes over me, I can't control it". An example of a danger meta-belief could be: "If I don't stop worrying soon, I'm going to lose my mind".

In addition, metacognitive beliefs about certain thoughts as particularly important, powerful and dangerous are described. An appraisal of the thought or impulse as harmful is then made. An example of this could be a person with OCD who believes that intrusive thoughts about harming someone are very dangerous and important to keep track of. These types of meta-beliefs about thoughts as important and dangerous are described in the model as fusion beliefs. Several types of fusion meta-beliefs occur in OCD: *Thought action fusion* (TAF), *thought event fusion* (TEF) and *thought object fusion* (TOF). Fusion beliefs are metacognitive beliefs that thoughts can influence events in the external world or that thoughts can be trans-ferred to objects in the external world. TAF is the idea that thoughts can make me do things I don't want to do. An example of TAF could be: "If I get an intrusive thought of sticking a kitchen knife into my partner's sto-mach, then the probability, the risk of me doing it, has suddenly increased". TEF is the belief that thoughts can cause negative events in the external world to occur. An example of TEF could be: "If I get the thought that my mother has been in a traffic accident, the risk increases that this has actually happened or will happen". TOF is the belief that thoughts can be transferred into external objects. An example of TOF could be: "I was wearing a pair of expensive new shoes when I got the news that my best friend had cancer. If I continue to wear the same shoes, I am putting myself and others at increased risk of cancer".

MCT is the only psychotherapy model that explains worry, rumination, and the other negative thought processes included in the concept of CAS, by dysfunctional metacognitive regulation and metacognitive beliefs. If MCT is a unique psychotherapy model in that way, what is the importance of that and what are the further implications? According to the model, the expla-natory power based on metacognition is significantly stronger. There is a wider range of psychological problems that become possible to explain and understand more precisely. In this way, it should also be possible to develop more effective and exactly targeted treatment interventions. Theoretically, MCT claims to be a new paradigm for psychological treatment. Problems with negative thinking such as worry and rumination, threat-focused atten-tion, as well as the behavioral strategies included in the concept of CAS, are of course not unknown phenomena in other psychotherapy models. In CBT, for example, similar cognitive and behavioral phenomena are usually explained by different schema models or by concepts from respondent and operant learning theories. Seen from the MCT perspective, these models provide weaker explanatory power. Schema models cannot explain exactly the process when an individual, based on a certain schema, engages in negative thought processes such as rumination and worry. Nor the process when that individual then interrupts the worrying/rumination. Even learning theories about respondent and operant conditioning through direct experi-ences/contingences, according to B.F. Skinner (1974), for example, are insufficient to explain human thinking/cognition. Many anxiety problems develop in the absence of clearly identifiable original aversive events or dis-tinguishable historical conditioning. The worry themes for patients with common psychological problems are often around events the individual has no previous direct experience of. For example, Mowrer's two-factor analysis of respondent and operant behavior has been criticized over the years (see, for example, Rachman, 1977). Mowrer's two-factor analysis can be con-sidered as highly insufficient in terms of explaining emotional problems where human thinking is involved, which really applies to most of the psy-chological problems that clients suffer from in clinical practice. Indeed, there are more recent developments of operant learning theories that aim to explain language and thinking (see, for example, Törneke, 2010, 2014). However, these do not seem to allow corresponding useful evidence-based explanations of mechanisms, or case formulations that in clear-cut ways inform the clinician about the targets for interventions and what the next step in the psychological treatment should be.

In several of the prominent contemporary CBT models, no clear distinction is made between trigger thoughts/negative automatic thoughts and negative thought processes such as worry and rumination; see for example Beck (2011). Whether MCT really provides more effective understanding and treatment is, of course, an empirical question. The predictions that can be made from the model are researchable. In Chapter 7, a detailed discussion of the current state of evidence for MCT as a theoretical model and as a treatment will follow.

In metacognitive therapy, the goal is to systematically reduce CAS and modify dysfunctional metacognition. Negative thoughts and negative emotions are assumed to be a part of life, a normal part of everyday life. "Thoughts don't matter but your response to them does", says the originator of MCT, Adrian Wells (Wells, 2009, p.1). According to MCT, we all have negative thoughts, and we also believe in them from time to time. It is not the negative thoughts that cause problems and that make us vulnerable, but how we relate to the thoughts. For example, both person A and person B could have a negative self-view. Person A often engages in the negative thoughts of himself. He organizes his life around these beliefs, avoids, for example, various challenges and certain social events. In addition, A thinks a lot about how he is perceived by others and tries to scan for any signs of dislike from others. Person B usually doesn't care about the negative thoughts about himself. B even finds himself forgetting this for long periods of time and in connection with daily activities and meetings. In addition, B has discovered that he can continue to converse with and take an interest in another person even if his thoughts of himself as inferior, boring or less intelligent come to mind. According to MCT, it is not the negative thoughts that create problems, but the response to them in the form of perseverative negative thinking styles such as worry and rumination.

In MCT, the therapist and client explore together whether it is possible to relate to negative thoughts as what they are, namely, thoughts and temporary inner events that can be allowed to come and go by themselves. We can spend much time or less time thinking about the problems we all have to face in our lives. More thinking is far from always helpful but rather the opposite. Much of the thinking in the case of mental illness can be characterized as repetitive, negative overthinking.

In MCT, compared to CBT's schema models where schema-restructuring is regarded as crucial, a negative self-view is not considered as some kind of inner permanent memory structure that needs to be changed. Instead, negative self-view is conceptualized as the conclusion that the individual can come to after persistent negative thinking. This means that individuals who refrain from prolonged engagement in negative thoughts about themselves, or only does so occasionally, will not suffer from the kind of problems commonly referred to as "self-esteem" or "negative self-image problems".

According to MCT, it is the prolonged response to negative thoughts that causes problems in our lives. The problems begin when we try to control these self-regulating systems of inner experiences, when we try to control thoughts and feelings instead of letting them self-regulate and come and go as temporary and passing internal events.

The S-REF model, the cognitive attentional syndrome CAS and metacognition

MCT is based on the S-REF-model (*self-regulatory executive function model*) (Wells & Matthews, 1994, 1996); see a simplified version of the S-REF model in Figure 2.1. The model delineates thoughts and thought processes on three different and interacting levels. The S-REF model describes cognitive and

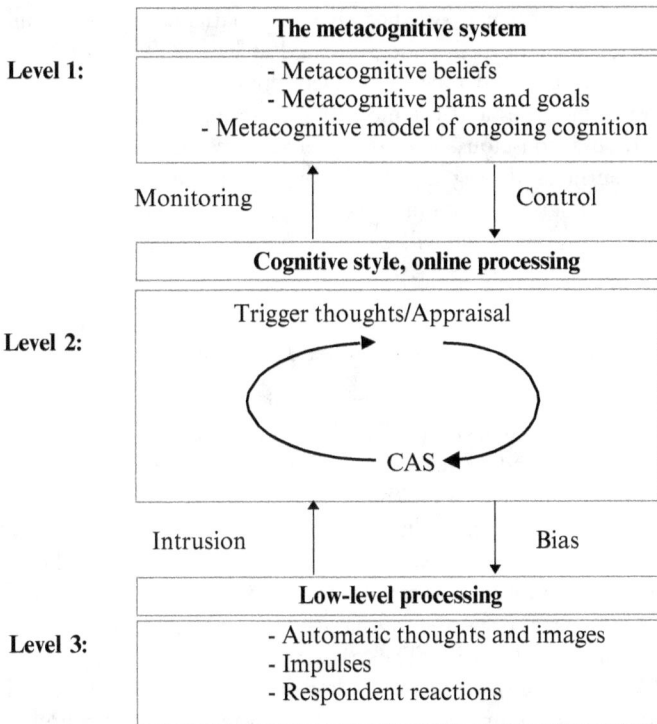

Figure 2.1 The S-REF model, simplified and adapted version, from *Attention and Emotion: A Clinical Perspective*, by Wells and Matthews © (1994) by Psychology Press. Reproduced by permission of the Taylor & Francis Group.

metacognitive factors involved in the perpetuation of emotional problems. It is a so-called top-down model that explains how top-level metacognition monitors and controls the thought processes and attention at the middle level (*online processing*), which in turn affects and is affected by the lowest level (*low-level processing*).

Level 3 in the S-REF: Low-level processing

Although the S-REF is a top-down model, let's start from the bottom with level 3, the automatic level. Low-level processing at this level means that sensory impressions and stimuli are processed automatically, outside volitional and conscious control.

Many sensations and sensory impressions never reach the conscious level, and information-processing then stays at and is never leavs level 3. Some of the processes at this level are conditioned respondent associations. For example, a person with OCD suffering contamination obsessions may, due to previous respondent learning, associate more stimuli in a bathroom with dirt and bodily secretions than individuals without similar problems. From level 3, trigger thoughts, i.e. negative automatic thoughts, impulses and images, arise, which can then be processed at level 2. Through CAS at level 2 and by the attentional focus selectively directed and biased towards possible threats, the threshold for more trigger thoughts or *intrusions* to reach the middle and conscious level is lowered. Anyone who is scanning contaminated surfaces during OCD will experience more frequent conscious trigger thoughts about contamination. Anyone who scans for experiences of dizziness in panic disorder will experience more trigger thoughts related to ongoing physiology.

Level 2 in S-REF: Cognitive style, online processing

The middle level of the model consists of so-called *online processing* or cognitive style. At this level, it is outlined how CAS, i.e. worry, rumination, threat monitoring and unhelpful behaviors, constitutes a response to negative automatic thoughts/trigger thoughts. The individual is "online", directly engaged in the negative thoughts. CAS is to be understood as metacognitive strategies, as coping strategies, in relation to a trigger thought. For example, if I should feel pain in my stomach and get the trigger thought "What if it's cancer!", CAS is a response to that thought and a goal directed coping strategy controlled by will. The trigger can be dealt with by continued worry: "What if I have to undergo a lot of painful examinations? How will my children cope if I am seriously ill?" Soon, the client may continue to scan their body for pain or new symptoms. Possibly the person spends many hours googling "pain in the stomach". Or the person asks a close relative if they think it could be something serious. It is not uncommon that the person also tries different ways to get distracted from the thoughts that by now may be experienced as very painful. Sometimes alcohol is used to reduce worry. In the previous example, worry is described as a main thought process. An equally important thought process is rumination. Rumination often revolves around "why-questions", i.e. rumination is not future-oriented in the same way as worry, and often the questions involve a repetitive introspective analysis of one's own feelings, motivation or different decisions made in the past. Again, CAS is to be understood as volitional coping strategies and as responses to the trigger thought. Additional CAS may also occur as strategies for dealing with worry and rumination, such as worry for worry or avoidance to reduce worry.

Level 1 in the S-REF: The metasystem

Metacognition is cognition applied to cognition. As mentioned earlier, the S-REF is a top-down model. This means that metacognition is the level that controls and monitors thinking and CAS, and indirectly also the processes at the lowest automatic level (low-level processing). Metacognition is the part of cognition that regulates thinking according to metacognitive goals. "How do you know and decide when to finish worrying?" is a question that can be asked to the client in MCT. It is an exploratory question regarding the metacognitive goals of worry and about the start and stop signals for the worry. Stop signals for worry can sometimes be emotional stimuli, such as "I worry until I feel calmer". Such a stop signal would of course be problematic since worry usually increases anxiety, which in turn then gives impetus to continue the worry process. Different beliefs the client has about their thoughts and thought processes are identified, examined and challenged in the treatment. There are both positive and negative metacognitive beliefs in the model. Positive metacognitive beliefs are beliefs about worry or rumination as helpful and protective strategies, for example "By worrying, I will protect my children from accidents". There are two kinds of negative metacognitive beliefs: Beliefs about CAS as uncontrollable or beliefs about CAS as dangerous to engage in. These two kinds of negative meta-beliefs, as well as coexisting positive meta-beliefs, tend to occur concurrently. A common example of a negative meta-belief about uncontrollability is "my worry is completely out of control". An example of a negative danger metacognitive belief could be "If I don't manage to stop worrying, I'm going to damage my brain and body with stress".

Among people with emotional and psychological problems, worry, rumination and other CAS activities are rarely experienced as voluntarily and controlled coping strategies. Rather, they are usually felt to be difficult to control thought processes and even as parts of the disorder and as symptoms. If one were to experience only benefits from worry and rumination, one would hardly be inclined to seek psychotherapeutic help. If one had the experience of worry and rumination only as painful and symptom-increasing phenomena, but at the same time easily controlled thought processes, it would be no point in continuing the CAS, and neither in a situation like that, would one be prone to seek help. It would be enough and easy, just to interrupt and end the negative thought processes. A person who is depressed often tends to believe that rumination is one of the depressive symptoms. Depressive rumination is often also believed to be the solution and the way to cure depression, although rumination at the same time is experienced as tiresome, painful and leading to increased pessimism. "I need to understand why I feel so down and dejected". The patient's experiences of worry and rumination as uncontrollable processes will, by the S-REF model, be identified as metacognitive beliefs of uncontrollability, i.e. as processes in the top level, the metasystem. To the extent that worry, and rumination are also experienced as harmful processes for one's own mind or body, this is identified as negative metacognitive beliefs about danger. Thus, even though CAS is conceptualized as coping strategies, these strategies are ineffective and even counterproductive. This makes the individual feel ineffective in their ability to regulate attention, thoughts and emotions. By that, negative metacognitive beliefs at level 1 will increase. It will often result in a feeling that one's own mind is a hostile and dangerous site. Ineffective mind control strategies increase negative metacognitive beliefs that worry is indeed both uncontrollable and dangerous.

If a person believes that they are protecting themselves from various dangers by worrying, it is of course understandable that the worry continues. The worry is thus driven by a positive metacognitive belief. Such a belief can be explored and challenged: "Are you really sure that you'll become safer and more secure by worrying? Because your reason for seeking therapy, isn't that related to anxiety problems and persistent feelings of insecurity?" If one believes that analyzing yourself and your depressive mood will help you find the cause of depression and thereby the solutions to it, a continued rumination process makes a lot of sense. Even such a metacognitive belief can be examined and challenged: "Has rumination so far worked in overcoming your depression or is it rather the case that the depression deepens when you dwell on things?" The following dialogue between patient (P) and therapist (T) is intended to illustrate how metacognitive beliefs can be identified at an initial stage of therapy:

P: I worried so much before the doctor's visit that I felt ready to cry, was nauseous and even started to worry about my mental health.

T: *That sounds like you were having a hard time and that it was quite exhausting for you. You worried not only about getting a serious message about your health, but also about the worry as such [Identifying so-called meta-worry]. Do you think your worry can be harmful? [Examines negative metacognitive beliefs about danger]*

P: I'm convinced of that. I've been exhausted before, and the worry makes me stressed and so tired.

T: *Okay, you're convinced that your worry can hurt you [sums up]. Did you try to reduce your worry? [Begins to explore metacognitive beliefs of worry as uncontrollable.]*

P: When I'm anxious and worry like that, nothing helps.

T: *You find it completely impossible to interrupt the worry in such situations?*

P: Then it just doesn't work.

T: *In addition to perceiving your worry as both harmful to your health and at times impossible to control, do you also have positive beliefs about it? [Examines positive metacognitive beliefs] Does the worry make you more prepared? Do you think it would be risky not to worry about your health?*

It's quite understandable how the worry will continue based on positive metacognitive beliefs. It is also conceivable how negative metacognitive beliefs imply continued worry or rumination. Anyone who experiences the worry as uncontrollable sees no reason to interrupt ongoing worry with sufficient determination. A notion here can often be "even if I could interrupt the worry now, it will come back later and then even much worse". Anyone who believes that rumination is controlled by biological processes finds it difficult to see the point of doing nothing with the negative thoughts and thus interrupting the rumination. Anyone who thinks that worry or rumination are thought processes that harm mental or physical health tends to worry about this rather than resolutely just interrupting the negative thought process. Metacognitive beliefs of worry/rumination as uncontrollable processes are linked to the danger meta-beliefs. Clients who experience worry and rumination as uncontrollable and problematic thought processes naturally also have perceptions of these, in some sense or other, as harmful and dangerous. Otherwise, the belief of uncontrollability would of course be perceived as completely unproblematic, as a non-issue.

A closer look at the S-REF model

We will return to the different levels of S-REF, now with an in-depth look at metacognition, the trigger–response relationship, different types of worry and rumination, appraisal of thoughts, the negative consequences of CAS and experience based on either object mode or metacognitive mode.

A closer look at level 1 in S-REF, the metasystem

Metacognition concerns goals, knowledge, strategies, experience, monitoring and control of cognition. One can compare the metacognitive level to both the score and the conductor of an orchestra. The metasystem is the level that monitors, evaluates and regulates so that cognition and attention are used according to goals and plans. The concept of metacognition is also used in educational psychology. Examples from that area could be: "Do I know the French vocabulary that is my homework assignment for tomorrow? How can I check that I know and how can I go about remembering them tomorrow as well?" From clinical psychology, the examples look a little different, for example: "In order to recover from my depression I need to remember and analyze my way to the point in life where things went awry" or "I need to carefully think through everything that could go wrong on this journey in order to be prepared to deal with different dangers and obstacles that might occur". A client in psychotherapy could hold the metacognitive belief "in order to be able to socialize with others, my mind must be free from negative thoughts and feelings". The metacognitive goal may then be to eliminate and reduce negative thoughts through various CAS strategies such as rumination, avoidance, thought suppression or alcohol. It is the metacognitive level of thinking that evaluates and controls whether the thought process leads forward according to the goal. In MCT, dysfunctional metacognition is regarded as more important than the processes referred to as CAS. Furthermore, negative meta-beliefs are assumed to be more problematic than the positive ones and are thus more prioritized to modify in psychotherapy. When a negative meta-belief of worry as an uncontrollable process has been modified through treatment into the belief and experience of worry as a completely controllable thought process, worry ceases to be a problem for the client. When an obsession in OCD or a trauma memory in PTSD is no longer perceived as a dangerous mental event that needs to be addressed or controlled, the thought is no longer perceived as scary.

Are some thoughts worse, bigger or more important?

Is there any difference between a thought of evil sudden death and a thought of a dessert with strawberries and ice cream? If so, how is the difference to be determined? The question is metacognitive, if what is being discussed is what we believe about cognitions and not pleasant, unpleasant, or even catastrophic events in the external world. Anyone who has finished eating strawberries with ice cream and at the same time is seriously dissatisfied with their weight, could start to worry intensely while their stomach feels too firm. A person who dreams of becoming a crime writer could imagine a story where frozen strawberries and ice cream become murder weapons, later to be eaten up, in a similar way to a frozen lamb roast in a short story by Roald Dahl. A question arises: How come some thoughts seem to become more persistent than others and harder to get rid of? Trying to figure that out, is a meta-cognitive exploration about appraisals and choices to relate to certain thoughts as more important than others. The questions in MCT can be: Who is it that evaluates and monitors your thoughts? How does the process look like when you categorize them as more or less important? Like big or small, innocent or dangerous? Can a thought really be big or dangerous at all? Does a thought become more important if you feel anxious at the same time? How do you decide if you are done with a certain line of thought and when it is time to leave it? The metacognitive system is the level of cognition that evaluates and categorizes thoughts, and that monitors and controls thought processes. Much of this monitoring and control takes place nonverbally. In MCT, a special conversation style, the metacognitive exploratory dialogue, is used to raise awareness of, and to examine and modify dysfunctional metacognition.

Level 2 and the trigger–response relationship

It's important to increase awareness of the trigger–response relationship. Trigger thoughts are those appearing spontaneously. They are often association-driven, and they are beyond volitional control. If we plan to do something difficult, it is almost surprising if the thought "what if I fail" does not appear. Anyone who has been in an accident and approaches the same situation again may have the thought "What if it happens again!" These are negative automatic thoughts, which indicate that they are not voluntary. They intrude from level 3 of the model. Thoughts are usually short lived and transient. That is, they are temporary if we do not continue to engage with them. According to MCT, the thoughts have no significance for our well-being and our functioning. It is not any special kind of negative thoughts that affect our well-being, nor the amount or frequency of them. What determines whether a thought takes on the character of a trigger is governed by meta-cognitive processes. Thoughts that for some reason are appraised as particularly important or threatening can be perceived as urgent to respond to and deal with. A person who suffers from anxiety or depression is unlikely to have any other trigger thoughts than people who experience mental well-being. If the person believes that certain thoughts are dangerous, such as a thought of harming someone, and at the same time experiences such an intrusive thought, this evaluation of the trigger is a metacognitive process. If the person then tries to push the thought away from consciousness, one can conclude that there is both a response to the trigger and an evaluation of it as dangerous. Trying to push thoughts away, trying to forget them, is described as thought suppression. Thought suppression thus constitutes a metacognitive strategy and a response to the trigger. Most often, the effect is paradoxical, that is, the thought returns or remains instead of vanishing and having appeared only as an ephemeral internal event.

Trigger thoughts can occur "embedded" in seemingly positive or neutral thoughts. For example, at the sight of a couple in love: "How happy they look!" Such a thought should not induce a negative emotional state, should it? Well, unless the next thought, that is, the trigger, becomes: "But what about me? Do I have any feelings for my boyfriend anymore?" Every moment in life and every thought can have an associative negative twist or rather be *given* a negative twist, for example, "What a lovely summer day!" can be followed by: "This day is actually unnaturally warm for the season.

How will my children be affected by climate change?" Another example could be the one who states, "Oh how happy I feel!" and then continues: "Before this occasion, when was really the last time I laughed? Why is it so rare that I seem to feel happy? Do I really live a happy life?"

If trigger thoughts arise spontaneously, involuntarily, association-driven and are also transient in nature, it's a different case with the CAS and repetitive negative thought processes. Negative thinking such as worry, and rumination are understood in MCT as volitional responses to trigger thoughts. To have a temporary thought about the risk of failing is something different from responding to and persistently engaging in that thought and in the following thoughts on that theme.

In MCT the focus will be on when and how the CAS is activated. Because CAS, together with dysfunctional metacognition, is understood as the cause of emotional problems and psychological disorders, it becomes important to find out how the CAS can be deactivated. When the client discovers the ability to refrain from or cancel the CAS at any time, then the negative metacognitive belief about worry/rumination as uncontrollable, will be reduced.

Given that CAS is conceptualized as a response to, and an engagement in the trigger, is it possible instead to "non-respond" or to "non-engage"? The non-response in relation to a trigger thought is captured in MCT with the concept *detached mindfulness* (DM). DM is an alternative, a new approach that the therapist and client will return to throughout the therapy. DM can be understood as the antithesis of CAS. A large part of the therapeutic interventions in MCT are centered around this type of non-response, and we will return to the therapeutic interventions in chapters 3 and 4. To illustrate how the exploration of the trigger and CAS can look like, what will follow is a fictive dialogue between patient (P) seeking help for anxiety problems and therapist (T):

T: *Would you like to tell me about the symptoms that have bothered you?*
   [Begins exploration at level 3]
P: Above all, it's severe anxiety in some situations that I consider should be unproblematic to manage for any normally functioning adult.
T: *Can you describe the last time you experienced something like this? When was it and what anxiety symptoms did you notice?*
P: Yesterday after a customer call. I felt shaky, dizzy, had a tightness in my chest and suddenly felt an urge to cry.
T: *When you noticed these symptoms, what might have been the first thought that came to your mind? [Starting to identify trigger thought at level 2]*
P: Hmm, the thought was probably something like "I'm losing it. I can't even manage to carry out regular customer conversations anymore".
T: *When that thought popped into your mind, what did you do with it? Did you just let it pass? Or did you continue to worry about your symptoms and what might happen to you if these reactions should continue? [Begins to explore worry as a CAS process, level 2]*

P: I started to worry about what's gone wrong with me, that I might not be able to do this job anymore and, if so, what then will happen.

T: *Did you do anything else with the thought? For example, did you start analyzing why the symptoms appeared and the reasons for them? Did you dwell on the reactions of those around you, whether the customer or your colleagues noticed your symptoms or whether they judged you in a negative way based on that? [Begins to explore the presence of rumination, level 2]*

P: I often think about what has made me so sensitive and what people around me really think of me.

T: *Did your attention change in any way? Did you become more vigilant about what was happening in your body and whether your physical symptoms continued to increase or began to decrease? [Begins to explore threat monitoring, level 2]*

P: In such situations, I become very focused on the dizziness and this unpleasant pressure in the chest. It becomes almost unbearable for me.

T: *What about your behavior, did you behave in any special way to cope with your symptoms? Did you stay where you were, or did you leave? [Examines behavioral responses to the trigger and behaviors intended to reduce worry or rumination.] Do you have any anti-anxiety medication that you usually take on similar occasions?*

P: What I then did was to use box breathing as I had previously learned. After that, I also called my partner wanting to hear a soothing voice.

The example above illustrates how the exploration of CAS in relation to symptoms and triggers can look within the framework of the metacognitive dialogue. A natural continuation in such a dialogue is then to explore dysfunctional metacognitive beliefs that control worry, rumination and other CAS activity. Somewhat later in the treatment, detached mindfulness will also be introduced and practiced, i.e. the principle of non-response to the trigger and symptoms.

What is worry? Type 1 and type 2 worry

Worry is defined as an inner verbal activity, as persistent chains of thought about negative future events that may occur, with the aim of problem-solving (Borkovec et al., 1983). Worry is engaging in thoughts about bad things that might happen. That is, there is a significant difference between having a spontaneous trigger thought about, for example having a terminal illness, and then engaging in that thought for prolonged periods of time, and in further thoughts about aversive consequences that could possibly then follow. In a similar way, there is a significant difference between having a spontaneous thought that you are a failure as a parent compared to responding to the trigger and engaging in thoughts about further negative consequences in the long run. A person who suffers from their worry and seeks help with it has often also developed worry about worry, so-called meta-worry or type 2 worry. In MCT, the term type 1 worry is used to describe worry about different bad things that can happen in life. Type 1 worry might be about accidents, illness, poor finances, being abandoned or rejected, etcetera. Type 2 worry is worry about the consequences of continued worry, for example: "What if the worry continues forever. What if I get a stroke from all the worry. What if my partner and friends get tired of me because I'm always so worried?"

Worry and anxiety are not synonymous concepts

In MCT and according to S-REF, a distinction is made between worry and anxiety. Worry is a CAS process, anxiety is not. Anxiety-related bodily sensations, such as palpitations or shortness of breath, belong to the lowest level, *low-level processing*. In everyday speech, the terms are often used synonymously, but in MCT and in some other psychological treatments, worry is defined as a negative future-oriented thought activity while anxiety is defined as a body sensations or an emotional state. Even in some clinical contexts, concepts such as "anticipatory anxiety" are used, but based on the discussion here, in MCT that would be conceptualized as worry. Obviously, you can also worry about your anxiety, which is very common in various anxiety disorders. When you worry, that is, start thinking intensely about various disaster scenarios, anxiety usually increases. In everyday life and using lay vocabulary (at least in Swedish), you can use the same word for worry ("oro") also when you are referring to restlessness or uncomfortable stomach sensations. In MCT you would then need to create greater clarity about the body sensation, distinguish it as a body sensation/feeling and then explore whether the person in question has any negative thoughts or catastrophic fantasies related to this. In an everyday conversation, you could also say "I feel so anxious about the meeting I'm going to have with my doctor". In MCT, you would explore whether it's rather worry that the person suffers from and how prolonged thinking about the coming meeting with the doctor results in increased fear and anxiety. The dialogue between the therapist (T) and patient (P) could then look something like this:

P: I feel so anxious about the medical examination.

T: *Do you worry about it?*

P: Well, I feel really scared. In fact, I'm so scared that I get nauseous and totally lose my appetite.

T: *What is it that scares you when you think about the medical examination?*

P: Obviously, they could find something bad and serious, such as cancer.

T: *How long have you been thinking that they might possibly find something serious?*

P: During the last week, almost all the time. Last week was tough and exhausting.

T: *There seems to have been a lot of thinking going on. Sounds like a lot of worry, doesn't it? What happens to your emotions and your anxiety when you persistently worry that you may receive bad news or have a serious illness? [The therapist by this dialogue makes a differentiation between anxiety and worry and further examines the emotional consequences of worry.]*

Rumination

Rumination is a similar repetitive negative thought process as worry. While worry often begins with the trigger thought "What if…" (something bad happens), rumination is often retrospective, overly self-analytical, and often begins with the thought "Why … ?" For example, "Why do I feel as bad as I do? Why don't I feel more joy? Why don't I feel interested? Why don't I see more meaning in my life?". Depressive rumination is characterized, according to *response style theory* (Nolen-Hoeksema, 1991, 2000), by the individual reacting to a negative mood by repeatedly immersing himself in the depressive symptoms. The rumination process can often also revolve around anger and the theme of injustice/perceived injustices. "It's not right that I am treated like this! I shouldn't be expected to put up with this." At other times, the rumination process may revolve around self-pity: "Why should I have to suffer like this? Haven't I already had enough setbacks and difficulties?"

Additional rumination themes can be guilt, such as: "Is person X disappointed in me without telling me? If so, what could I have said or done? Didn't he look disappointed the last time we met?" Or about shame: "Why am I so confined, stiff and restrained at social gatherings? They must think I'm uninteresting, odd and socially unattractive."

A special form of rumination is referred to in MCT *as gap-filling*, and this involves a repetitive review of memories and a search for memory gaps in them. "How exactly did I say that to person Y and how did they react?" Gap-filling often occurs in post-traumatic stress disorder (PTSD), for example: "When exactly did I discover the other driver before the collision? What did I do the seconds before that?"

In addition, it is not entirely uncommon for clients in the therapy situation to express a form of meta-rumination: "Why don't I stop this rumination?! Why do I always have to ruminate like this?"

Ruminating together: Co-rumination

Rumination usually occurs as an inner persevering dialogue but can also appear in external dialogues (for an overview, see for example Spendelow et al., 2017), in friendships, in the workplace, in couple relationships, between parent and child or between client and psychotherapist. Co-rumination between client and therapist should of course be seen as a highly problematic and counterproductive process, and something very important for the therapist to recognize, pay attention to, label and intervene on.

Doubt

Doubting is universal but doubt also occurs as repetitive negative thinking and can take the form of worry or rumination, i.e. CAS. "Did I lock the door a few moments ago or did I not? Do I feel something genuine for my partner anymore or has all love died between us? Does she still love me, or does she just reassure me without being honest? Should I quit this workplace and change jobs?" Persistent doubts can exist as either worry or rumination or both. Examples of worry can be: "Did I lock the door or what if our apartment is still unlocked, someone gets in, and it turns out to be my fault?" "Should I stay where I am or what if I waste my life staying in this workplace?" Examples of rumination and gap-filling, attempts to fill gaps in memory, can be: "Did it really click in the lock when I locked the door or does my memory deceive me?"

Self-blame and a self-punishing inner dialogue

Self-blame, self-accusations and a self-punishing inner dialogue often occur as negative repetitive thought processes (Jannati et al., 2020; Kolubinski et al., 2016) and as common CAS activity in depressive disorders, personality disorders and further in a range of emotional problems where negative self-image (Fearn et al., 2022; Kolubinski et al., 2019) is evident in therapy. "Why can't you do anything right!? You idiot, you don't deserve anything better!?", "How could you be so stupid that you imagined him to be attracted to you!?" Of course, a recurring self-punishing inner dialogue affects the self-regulation of emotions and cognition and has similar negative consequences as worry and rumination. A self-punishing inner dialogue, repetitive self-blame can be conceptualized as a variant of rumination.

Suicidal rumination

Suicidal rumination has been identified as a risk factor for later suicidal acts and even completed suicide. Mapping of suicidal thoughts is usually recommended in suicide risk assessments in psychiatry practice, but assessment of suicidal rumination is probably even more important, i.e. how often, for how long and how intensely the involvement in suicidal thoughts occurs. Suicidal rumination increases the incidence of suicidal thoughts. The term *suicidal ideation* is not clearly operationalized, and no clear distinction is made there between suicidal thoughts and prolonged suicidal thinking; see, for example, Harmer et al. (2021).

Pelle is a psychologist at a psychiatric outpatient clinic. In his office, he meets clients every week where he needs to do risk assessments. He makes these assessments according to the clinic's guidelines and he asks questions about the client's experiences of meaninglessness, boredom of life, suicidal thoughts and suicidal intentions or plans. Pelle knows that many of the clinic's clients have suicidal thoughts, and he also knows that it is extremely difficult, even with structured assessment instruments, to predict who will later carry out suicidal acts and who will not. This time, when he meets his client Olle, Pelle is aware that it is probably rather suicidal rumination that constitutes a risk factor than the presence of suicidal thoughts. Pelle strives to help Olle reduce suicidal rumination and thus reduce the risk of suicidal acts.

PELLE: *Would it be okay for you to tell me a bit more about your thoughts on ending your life?*

OLLE: I've been thinking a lot about it the last few days. I have a lot of anxiety. I can hardly stop thinking about it. The thoughts haunt me. At the same time, I think that if I die, I will be free from thoughts and all anxiety. It would probably also be better for my family in the long run.

PELLE: *I understand that you have a hard time with these thoughts and that you find it difficult to leave them alone. Could one say you are dwelling or ruminating on the question of whether you have the strength to live on or not?*

OLLE: Yes, one can probably say it's rumination, but it's not something that I choose to think about. Like I said, I can't escape the thoughts even when I try to.

PELLE: *Probably most adults can have these kinds of thoughts in difficult moments of life and when one can't see any way out. Would thoughts of death continue to be a problem if you discovered that it's possible not respond to them, not engaging in them?*

OLLE: It really doesn't feel like I can just ignore the difficult thoughts …

PELLE: *We can come back to that and further explore whether it is possible not to engage with them. It seems that all this worry and rumination about whether you should be able to live on makes you even more discouraged, anxious and depressed, and that the rumination consequently also leads to more thoughts of death. What you have tried so far does not seem to have reduced your thoughts. If you were to realize that there are effective strategies to radically reduce the worry and rumination around this theme, what would that mean for you?*

OLLE: Oh, that would make a huge difference and be a big relief, of course, but that sounds way too good to be true.

PELLE: *Shall we try for a moment an experiment that may help you discover that you have complete control over your rumination and that you can interrupt it whenever you like to? [Pelle and Olle carry out one of the experiments later described in chapters 3 and 4 of the book.]*

Rogers and Joiner (2018) found, among several risk factors, that suicidal rumination appeared to be the strongest risk factor for later suicidal action in a non-clinical sample (n = 300) of students. Rogers, Gallyer and Joiner (2021) found among 91 adults with a high suicide risk, that rumination over suicidal thoughts appeared to constitute a proximal risk factor for suicide. Wang et al. (2020) found among 894 college students that rumination was a mediating factor for the association between negative life events and suicidal thoughts, i.e. only during a high degree of rumination did suicidal thoughts after negative life events increase. Rogers, Gorday and Joiner (2021) found among 558 adults that, compared to the frequency, thought content and duration of suicidal rumination, the experience of suicidal rumination as uncontrollable was the strongest predictor of future suicide attempts. That is, based on the S-REF model, even if not explicitly mentioned in their paper, a plausible interpretation would be that the authors identified a metacognitive uncontrollability belief as a strong risk factor. Based on the S-REF model, suicide may be perceived as a possible solution for an individual who is in intense despair and who at the same time experiences the suicidal rumination as painful, frightening and uncontrollable. In a clinical sample of 24 participants, Hallard et al. (2021) examined, among other things, rumination, self-punishing inner dialogue, worry, and thought suppression, using momentary sampling measures of thought activity (*experience sampling method*). They found that both rumination and other thought control strategies predicted suicidal thinking and that metacognitive beliefs predicted self-punishing thinking.

Desire thinking

In addition to worry and rumination, desire thinking (Spada, Caselli & Wells, 2013) has been studied as another form of perseverative thinking style, important when conceptualizing addictive behaviors; see for example Caselli and Spada (2015) and Mansueto, Martino et al. (2019). Desire thinking has been described as a style of thinking involving the "positive elaboration" of a craved target (Caselli & Spada, 2010). The craved target can be an activity, an object or a state. Correspondingly to worry and rumination as forms of repetitive thinking in response to trigger thoughts, desire thinking is a response to cravings, which are understood as intrusive "wanting" experiences from the automatic low-level processing in the S-REF. Desire thinking involves the conscious and voluntary processing of the pleasant consequences of attaining the desired target and the planning of how to attain it. Desire thinking is thus conceptualized as a conscious and voluntary cognitive process orienting to prefigure images, information and memories about positive target-related experience. Desire thinking seems to be multi-dimensional in nature, with imaginal prefiguration and verbal perseveration components (Caselli & Spada, 2011). The imaginal prefiguration refers to positive imagery, anticipating the target with multi-sensory elaboration or recalling positive target-related memories. The verbal perseveration component refers to planning and to prolonged self-talk regarding worthwhile reasons for engaging in target-related activities and their achievement.

Desire thinking has been found to increase confidence in *permissive beliefs* in alcohol cravings (Caselli et al., 2021). Furthermore, in longitudinal studies, desire thinking has been found to predict cravings and binge drinking (Martino et al., 2017) and relapse after treatment (Martino et al., 2019). It has been found to be present across different addictive behaviors (Mansueto, Martino et al., 2019). Desire thinking can also be considered as a potential therapeutic target in compulsive sexual behaviors (Olivari et al., 2025), problematic internet pornography use (Allen et al., 2017), gambling disorder (Chen, Spada et al., 2024) and in problematic video game use (Bonner et al., 2022).

The role of attention in emotional regulation, threat monitoring

If you really pay attention to it for a while, it is usually possible to find potential life hazards wherever you are right now. External and internal disasters can of course occur at any time. Anyone who actively keeps an eye out for possible threats will become aware of more potential dangers. Those who are busy looking for threats and dangers will at the same time find it hard to relax, enjoy life and to focus on other tasks. In MCT, the concept of threat monitoring refers to how prolonged and biased attention to potential upcoming dangers occurs in most forms of emotional problems and psychological disorders. Threat monitoring can be directed to external dangers, such as hostile intentions of other people, but also to internal threats. Those who are bothered by mental illness often experience certain thoughts, memories, feelings and body sensations as threatening. Even the absence of discomfort can sometimes be perceived as something threatening, for example: "Why does everything feel so calm? Have I been off guard? Have I missed considering something important? Is this the calm before the storm?"

A depressed person can for long periods of time scan for lacking motivation or for the absent feeling of being interested or just a little more alert. What follows is a hypothetical dialogue to explore threat monitoring in a depressed patient:

P: I couldn't get out of bed all morning. I felt completely exhausted and empty inside.

T: *Could you describe this feeling of being completely exhausted and empty a bit more?*

P: As if all the energy had left me and as a total joylessness and meaninglessness.

T: *When you were lying there in bed, what did you pay attention to? Mostly to external stimuli, towards your surroundings or mainly towards internal events?*

P: My attention was almost only self-focused.

T: *Did you scan your fatigue?*

P: Yes, I tried to determine how tired I really was and whether I would be able to get up.

T: *What happened to your energy when you scanned and tried to assess your fatigue?*

P: I didn't get any more alert. Rather, even more exhausted.

T: *How do you determine the difference between having enough and insufficient energy to get up? Is there a particular feeling in your body that you are looking for?*

P: That was a difficult question. I guess it can vary from day to day.

T: *You also said that you experienced joylessness. Were you searching for a sense of joy?*

P: Yes, and I realized that it had been a very long time since I felt happiness.

T: *When you scan for joy and joylessness in that way, what happens to your depression?*

The thought processes worry, and rumination could also be understood in terms of attention allocation, i.e. certain negative thoughts are paid attention to very often and for extended periods of time. "Gap-filling rumination" could be understood as persistent threat monitoring of memory images, or rather of the gap between them, the memory gaps. "What does it mean when I don't remember the exact sequence of events?" Worry could be described as a persistent scan of catastrophic fantasies: "Have I now imagined and considered everything that could go wrong?" The scan, the worry/rumination process, can also be based on bodily sensations: "I still feel tense and anxious, does that mean that something is wrong in my life?" When people describe the best moments in life, they often refer to states when they have forgotten themselves and felt in connection with their environment, other people and the activity they have been engaged in. Much of the research on the relation between attention and emotion indicates that attention instead of being external, tends to become self-focused in the case of mental illness (see e.g. Ingram, 1990).

In previous psychological models of mental disorders, it has often been assumed that attention is regulated automatically, for example in various anxiety reactions. The S-REF model and MCT are based on more recent knowledge of the relationship between attention and emotion, which shows that attention is to a very large extent under volitional control and that it is governed by metacognition, i.e. by metacognitive beliefs, goals, monitoring and strategy choices (Wells & Matthews, 1994). Anyone who holds positive metacognitive beliefs about scanning for potentially dangerous people in a crowd will of course turn their gaze towards such stimuli. The monitoring for hostile people is likely to continue until the metacognitive goals are achieved or until something else is deemed more urgent to pay attention to. If a metacognitive goal could be formulated as "until I am absolutely sure that no person in this crowd has evil intentions", the goal will of course be very difficult to achieve, and the threat monitoring will thus continue. If you are engaged in similar threat monitoring, what data will be paid attention to? Many people in the environment may walk around with backpacks and bags where a weapon or an explosive device could be hidden. Someone looks tense, someone else may look grim or nervous. How do you form an opinion about the intentions of others? Maybe it's the one who looks totally calm and relaxed, perhaps even friendly, perhaps the one who thus shows a poker face, who has truly diabolical intentions? This type of problem could be encountered by a person with GAD or PTSD. Often, interoceptive data are made important in similar situations, for example: "I feel so tense and scared now, something is not right." Threat monitoring increases the feeling of anxiety and insecurity, feelings that in turn can be noticed by the meta-cognitive system that gives new "instructions": "Keep scanning, keep worrying!" Similar monitoring could be interrupted if I suddenly hear someone calling my name, turning around and seeing a friend happily waving.

Anyone who scans the heart rate to check if it appears abnormal is likely to become more aware of any possible arrhythmic in the pulse, and those who look for memories of past failures in their life will remember more of them. The S-REF model stipulates that threat monitoring, a process that is controlled by the metacognitive system, leads to a lowered threshold for certain stimuli to reach consciousness, for example for certain threat-related thoughts or bodily sensations. Through this "lowering of the threshold", more threat-related thoughts and sensations will intrude on consciousness. A person who is bothered by social anxiety thus becomes more aware of all facial expressions in the environment that could be interpreted as critical, or about how ridiculous your own voice can sound. Anyone who suffers from fear of flying becomes more aware of all the sounds and movements in the fuselage that could signal possible technical problems.

Unhelpful thought control and behavior strategies

The last element of CAS deals with counterproductive thought control or behavioral strategies. These include avoidance, flight, safety behaviors and the use of alcohol or other substances. These behaviors are understood as metacognitive strategies, aimed at dealing with trigger thoughts, but above all, the goal is to reduce worry or rumination by thought control and behavioral strategies.

Common examples of thought control strategies are thought suppression, i.e. trying to push unwanted thoughts out of consciousness. Think of exactly anything you want, except for a pink rabbit! The phenomenon is sometimes referred to as *the rebound effect*, i.e. when we try to push away thoughts, they tend to bounce back, and we get even more engaged with them. Usually, most of us don't think about pink rabbits at all. Thought suppression is also experienced as tiresome and at times even mentally exhausting. In clinical contexts, the thoughts dealt with by thought suppression tend to be different and are perceived as more threatening than those about pink rabbits. Another form of thought-control strategy is excessive reasoning, such as: "What indicates that this pressure on the chest could be something serious? What speaks against it?" Exaggerated reasoning can of course also take the form of repetitive rumination.

It is not uncommon to try to distract yourself with other behaviors or with other thoughts, and even then, you can see a paradoxical effect as in thought suppression. One can define distraction as always occurring together with an element of thought suppression. The goal of distraction is to shut out certain thoughts, to eliminate them from conscious mind. Through this, distraction is of course also a response to the trigger thought. To distract oneself or to engage in thought suppression is to simultaneously stay in contact with the thoughts, to relate to them and to make them important.

Unhelpful behavioral strategies for dealing with negative thoughts and thought processes often manifest themselves through various forms of avoidance. Anyone who worries about not feeling relaxed when arriving at the party to which they are invited, can choose not to go there. Avoidance then becomes a strategy to regulate worry. An individual who worries about not aiming for higher education may choose to stay in bed for the rest of the morning instead of getting ready and leaving home for class. Anyone who worries about being blamed for his opinion becomes anxiously restrained and withheld.

Other common ways to try to eliminate negative thoughts from consciousness or to reduce negative thought processes are using alcohol, illegal drugs/substances or legal prescription substances.

Individuals who experience various forms of anxiety usually recognize themselves in asking loved ones for reassurance, which is trying to regulate their own worries with the help of other people. A negative consequence is that confidence in one's own abilities is eroded. Another consequence is that relatives easily find the reassurance-seeking tiresome and that the relationship thus becomes more strained or unnecessarily asymmetrical. The possible calm that may arise after receiving reassurance from a loved one is usually short-lived.

Individuals suffering from obsessive-compulsive disorder use different cleansing rituals or other control rituals to deal with obsessive thoughts and negative thought processes. The rituals are performed with the aim of neutralizing/eliminating thoughts or doubtful thoughts such as "Am I really completely clean now? Did I lock the door, or did I not lock it?" The rituals can also be aimed at reducing worry, for example: "If I don't check that the electrical appliances are properly turned off one more time before I leave the house, I will worry about it for the rest of the day". One of the problems with similar rituals is that there is always room for more doubt: "Do I really remember correctly, did I really see correctly if I now decide that the stove is turned off?" Another very central problem, obviously, is that thoughts of being contaminated cannot be washed away with soap and water. Neither can an extra check of the stove be an effective way to prevent the intrusion of new thoughts that the stove still may be turned on. Ineffective and counterproductive coping strategies will strengthen beliefs that worry and rumination are uncontrollable thought processes. In addition, other meta-cognitive beliefs that thoughts are important, powerful and dangerous are easily reinforced, for example: "Even though I have put so much energy into trying to get rid of the obsessive thought of harming others, the thought persists. It must mean that the compulsion is stronger than I am and that it indeed is dangerous. Maybe it tells something important and true about the person I am. Perhaps, deep down inside, I want to harm others or cause a fire by leaving the stove plates on?"

Negative consequences of the CAS

Several negative consequences of CAS have already been outlined. The key is that CAS is to be seen as transdiagnostic factors in general and as causing mental illness and emotional problems. In two later chapters, chapters 5 and 6, CAS and metacognition will be described in a wide range of common disorders and emotional problems. From the preceding paragraphs, it also becomes obvious that CAS behaviors such as massive avoidance, over-consumption of alcohol, social isolation or compulsive rituals lead to new problems. The following paragraphs further examine the negative con-sequences of worry and rumination in terms of reduced possibilities for recovery and rest, concentration, self-reliance, emotion regulation and satis-fying interpersonal relationships.

Consequences of worry

Even though CAS is understood as coping strategies, their effect is para-doxical. The strategies are ineffective or directly counterproductive for the regulation of emotion and cognition. Between the three levels of the S-REF model, there is a mutual influence. Metacognitive processes con-trol CAS, but as CAS involves ineffective regulation, the experience of worry as an uncontrollable or dangerous thought activity increases. Since worry, rumination and threat monitoring could be considered as a long-term relationship to mental threat scenarios, it becomes difficult to relax and more difficult to feel interest and desire for life's small and big joys and for commitment to other projects and responsibilities. Those who are bothered by worry often also have problems with various bodily tensions. When you feel unsafe and insecure, it becomes difficult to focus on work tasks or on leisure activities like reading a book or watching a movie. Repeated and prolonged catastrophic thinking naturally increases and prolongs emotions such as fear and anxiety. Persistent worry also often leads to depression and depressive symptoms. Worry and rumina-tion are tiresome, resource-demanding mental processes. A person who is tired after spending hours with negative thinking easily becomes irritable. Most clients experience repetitive negative thinking as exhausting.

A person who feels tired of the worry sometimes continues to worry about the fatigue and the symptoms of exhaustion. The worry makes it much more difficult to find rest, relaxation and recovery. It's hard to calm down, fall asleep or go back to sleep with thoughts running wild. Evolution has shaped us to become creatures that do not sleep if a danger lurks in our vicinity. If stress is understood as relating to something that is perceived as threatening, i.e. what usually activates the so-called fight-flight response in humans and animals, it is of course also stressful to engage in repetitive, threat-focused thought- and attentional activity. The S-REF model explains why anxiety and stress follow from CAS and turn into persistent emotional problems.

Consequences of rumination

In a similar way that worry leads to a variety of negative consequences, rumination leads to emotional, cognitive and interpersonal problems. Rumination seems to be one of the most important factors behind depression (see, e.g., McLaughlin & Nolen-Hoeksema, 2011; Wilkinson et al., 2013). To persistently and repeatedly analyze why you feel the way you feel or why you have failed at certain things in life can easily turn into a negative spiral towards increasing depression. The rumination can also take the form of harsh self-accusations, where the tone of voice and comments in the inner dialogue are almost to be described as verbal harassment or "self-bullying". Cognitive side effects occur in the way that the memory of one's own or others' actions in social situations is distorted after a few days of rumination. Other people may be surprised and find it difficult to recognize themselves in the depiction of a social encounter that the person who has been ruminating intensely later reproduces. To ruminate on injustice or others' dishonesty is to perpetuate and cultivate anger. To ruminate on oneself as a defective social being is to cultivate shame and feelings of inferiority and alienation. To ruminate over any mistakes made is to cultivate feelings of guilt. To ruminate on whether the partner is telling the truth when she claims that she loves me and is faithful to me, is to cultivate jealousy, suspicion and a persistent fear of separation and abandonment. Not uncommon is an increasing and violent anger in the person who, after a period of rumination, feels convinced of the partner's falsehood.

Interpersonal problems resulting from worry and rumination

After worry and rumination follow interpersonal consequences. The individual who repeatedly worries can often be perceived as annoying with their worry-driven conversations and questions. The person who worries or ruminates tends to relate to their own thoughts instead of to the people around them. The one who ruminates tends to become more self-occupied and reserved. It is not uncommon for a person who is depressed to isolate themselves and withdraw so as to have enough time to ruminate and analyze themselves and their situation. Anyone who ruminates about injustice or possible dishonesty, often appears prickly, reserved and irritable in the eyes of others, sometimes as moody. Anyone who ruminates or worries and is occupied by jealousy often shows an interaction style that by others is perceived as controlling, guarding and suffocating. Anyone who worries or ruminates about their own believed inferiority can, in interaction with others, sometimes appear excessively submissive, sometimes excessively compensatory, self-assertive, or even condescending. To ruminate means that attentional resources are used inflexibly. The person who ruminates is often perceived as negative in their attitude to life and can appear bitter, rigid and sometimes unpleasantly cynical in the eyes of others. Despite the interpersonal problems that result from worry and rumination, the MCT therapist does not intervene directly on these, but instead against the negative thought processes that cause relationship problems.

Worry and rumination lead to more worry and rumination

The S-REF model stipulates that CAS are counterproductive strategies when dealing with stress, i.e. they backfire and cause even more and sustained stress. A person who worries a lot often gets something new to worry about: "What if my worries ruin my life, my health, if I due to that will lose my abilities to take care of my marriage, my family or my job? What if I make my children feel insecure and transfer my worries to them?" If you try to reduce your worry related to social situations by avoiding them, even more social situations will likely appear scary and possible to worry about. If you choose extreme social isolation as an avoidance strategy, you can soon start to worry about situations like meeting a neighbor in the hallway or having to make an everyday phone call. A person who excessively monitors how they can be perceived in the eyes of others becomes less listening, more absent and finds it more difficult to establish natural contact with others. If you don't accept challenging tasks in life because of worry for failure, many learning opportunities will get lost as well as chances for personal development, which then can appear as new themes for worry and rumination as well as reinforced perceived incompetence. Anyone who repeatedly tries to reduce worry or rumination with alcohol, sooner or later develops alcohol-related problems to further keep worrying about.

Impaired self-confidence

Given that the CAS strategies are ineffective and may even backfire, a sense of general incompetence will often follow and more specifically, an impaired confidence regarding one's abilities to regulate emotion and cognition. Impaired self-confidence is understood in MCT as thoughts, and these cognitions are to be understood as conclusions and as the result of rumination and worry. People with long-term worry problems can express deep uncertainty about their own capacity to deal with the future, perfectly normal difficulties and challenges that life brings. For example, about the ability to cope with the inevitable aging and death of parents, or the responsibilities and trials that naturally come with parenthood. "What if I'm not going to be emotionally stable enough?" Some do not use their full potential in professional life due to lack of confidence in their own abilities. "If I were to accept that managerial job, what if I'm not able to deal with the different kinds of conflicts that will naturally occur in a workplace and that one is expected to handle in such a position? What if I don't manage to deal with others' needs? What if I don't have the strength, courage and energy required?" Anyone with the habit of asking others for reassurance finds that their trust in their own competence is eroded. Likewise, self-confidence regarding abilities to self-regulate decreases in those who use chemical substances when trying either to get rid of trigger thoughts or to reduce worry and rumination. Feeling entangled in your own thoughts is quite often a consequence of prolonged and intensive rumination. For example, when gap-filling and after trying to access clearer memories for the hundredth time, uncertainty will increase. Individuals who engage in similar rumination easily conclude that they have memory deficits and that they cannot trust their cognitive functions and their own mental apparatus. A person who has repeatedly engaged in doubts – "Did I turn off the stove or did I not?" – can, in addition to memory, easily also begin to doubt his five senses and his understanding. "Do I really see correctly now when I perceive that the stove is off?" Self-critical rumination together with dysfunctional metacognition has been shown to be predictive of negative self-image (Fearn et al., 2022; Kolubinski et al., 2019). It is not uncommon for those who are bothered by long-term worry problems also doubt whether their own intellectual level and general knowledge are sufficient and can be trusted. If I have out of habit related to trigger thoughts and anxiety as if they were relevant and important sources of information, the conclusion can easily be: "Admittedly, I have heard and read that it is almost completely harmless to fly, but my anxiety tells me otherwise." People who seek psychotherapy can sometimes say things like: "I'm the kind of person who can't say no", "I can't ride the subway when I am anxious", "I can't talk in front of a group of people", "I can't get out of bed if I feel unmotivated and depressed". Rather than a lack of competence/knowledge, the implicit meaning of similar statements is usually something like "In order to be prepared to carry out similar actions, my mind first needs to be clean and free from negative thoughts and from feelings that I could perceive as negative". That is, instead of a lack of energy, courage or competence in a person who experiences anxiety/depression, similar statements can be understood as governed by metacognitive beliefs about the meaning and importance of negative thoughts. The starting point in MCT is that the client usually does not have problems with skill deficiencies, but that self-confidence problems are instead to be conceptualized as the consequence of worry and rumination.

A way to describe it could be that information processing and knowledge acquisition seems to be based on recirculated thoughts instead of empirical data. Much of the CAS activity, such as for example many forms of avoidance, implies not exposing one's own beliefs/hypotheses to empirical testing against reality. If a person who arrives in a new city in a new country stays in his hotel room and tries to guess what the surroundings and opportunities look like, the thinking and guessing could go on forever, without any new knowledge being acquired.

Schema, intolerance of uncertainty, neuroticism, inflated responsibility, and perfectionism explained by the CAS and dysfunctional metacognition

As reviewed in the previous paragraphs, a negative self-view and negative view of the world around us – phenomena that are defined as schemas in several other CBT models – are conceptualized as consequences of repetitive negative thinking, in the S-REF model. Such conclusions about self and others can in turn appear as new trigger thoughts. In several CBT models, similar thoughts are given an explanatory value in the case of emotional problems, while according to the S-REF model they are understood as products of the CAS. Other cognitive constructs such as intolerance to uncertainty (Freeston et al., 1994), inflated responsibility (Salkovskis, 1985) or perfectionism (for a meta-analysis, see e.g. Limburg et al., 2017) are correspondingly also to be seen as additional thought content, by-products and consequences of CAS and dysfunctional metacognition. Perfectionism can, for example, be a theme for worry and rumination and perfectionist behaviors can serve as a strategy to regulate worry. Rumination may have elements of self-critical themes, and overzealous, perfectionist behaviors aim to reduce worry and rumination. Self-critical rumination and dysfunctional metacognition have been shown to mediate the relationship between perfectionism and problems with self-esteem (Fearn et al., 2022). Additional concepts such as neuroticism and *trait anxiety*, which have been considered as vulnerability factors for anxiety and depression, can be understood in the light of metacognition as underlying mechanism factors (Nordahl et al., 2019). See also Chapter 7 on evidence for the theoretical model and how these cognitive concepts seem to be better explained by the S-REF model.

Different ways of experiencing, in object mode and metacognitive mode

The S-REF model differentiates between experiences at the object level and at the metacognitive level. Much of the time we do not experience our thoughts as just thoughts but rather as perceptions or facts about ourselves and the world. According to MCT terminology, our experience in those moments is in object mode. When we think about a particular problem, that problem is the object of our thought activity. "How am I going to cope with my tasks at work today?" We are probably not even aware that it is thought activity we are performing or that the thoughts are separate from the physical objects in our environment. We may not be aware of the thoughts about the work situation as clearly separated from the physical work situation itself. We are experiencing at the object level when we cognitively process and try to deal with a problem in the external world. We are at the same time "online", that is, at an ongoing level of processing the problem in the external world. "By the way, where did I put the car keys?" could be a thought that suddenly intrudes into our consciousness as we are preparing to leave for work. When we make ourselves aware that we are thinking "now I'm thinking about work again, but I'm actually not there yet", we can have a more distinct experience of the thought as separate from the object. If, a moment later, a new thought should arise, such as "by the way, how can I manage to remember where I put the car keys?", we have moved to a metacognitive level and to the beginning of exploring metacognitive strategy choices. When cognition becomes the object of cognition, we can describe it as metacognition and our experience is then in metacognitive mode. All interventions in MCT are delivered from the metacognitive mode. Verbal techniques and various forms of metacognitive behavioral experiments are used to identify the old unhelpful ways of relating to thoughts and thought processes and to discover and try out new and more effective strategies.

Nelson (1996) shows how a postulated meta-level, a division between the object level and the meta-level, implies a solution to the so-called "Comte's paradox". Auguste Comte was a nineteenth-century philosopher, the founder of positivism, who, among other things, formulated a logical dilemma about self-reflection and consciousness: How can the same organ that observes also be the organ that is observed? How can both the instrument and the object of study be the same? Nelson describes how the object level and the meta-level, cognition and meta-cognition, can operate at the same time as interacting systems. By assuming a meta-level and an object level, the observer and the observed do not become completely identical, but rather as interacting systems.

Nelson also describes a theoretically possible model for how two general information flows can be created between the metacognitive level and the object level. Information about the status of the cognitive level flows to the metacognitive level through processes described as monitoring, such as, for example "I didn't understand that". Instructions from the meta-level to the cognitive level are delivered through control processes. This means that if cognitive errors occur at the object level, monitoring processes will make the meta-level aware, and control processes from the meta-level will be activated to correct the cognitive error, for example "Read the sentence again, but this time a bit slower!" The meta-level is also assumed to include a model that involves both goals and strategies for how the meta-level can use the object level to achieve the goal.

Typical clinical examples of experiences from object mode and metacognitive mode can be a statement such as "I am such a stiff and boring person". Such a statement is often perceived as a fact by those who describe this as a problem. Through the therapeutic dialogue in MCT, that experience is switched up to metacognitive mode, which means that the therapist through examining questions tries to identify and investigate thoughts about being stiff and boring and how such thoughts are dealt with by the individual. The metacognitive questions can then be: What do you do when you have such thoughts about yourself? Do you start worrying? Do you continue to ruminate over them/analyze yourself? Are you trying to cope with the thoughts in any way? Your feeling of being stiff and boring: Do you think it decreases or increases if you engage with your thoughts, and if you make them important? Do you become socially interactive, more open or less open to others when you engage with the thoughts that you are stiff and boring? Here is an example of how the therapist tries to switch up the dialogue from the object level to the metacognitive level with a depressed patient:

P: It feels like most decisions I've made so far in my life have been faulty and thoughtless. I have let my family down. Chosen work instead of being there for them when they would have needed me. I mean nothing to them anymore and I have no one to blame but myself.

T: *How often do you think along these lines?*

P: All the time.

T: *You've spent a lot of time thinking about this. What happens to you emotionally when you think about previous mistakes and letting your family down?*

P: I feel miserable, sad and angry with myself.

T: *Could you have been thinking enough about that? Is there anything that will get better if you keep thinking about it?*

Other examples of problems phrased from an object-level experience can be "I have severe problems with panic disorder". Questions that facilitate a shift to dialogue at the metacognitive level can then be: Do you often think about panic attacks? What are the thoughts you usually have during a panic attack and how do you usually relate to those thoughts? Do you usually worry about having new panic attacks or that they will get worse? Are you scanning for early signs that panic is coming? If you worry or scan panic, does the likelihood of new anxiety attacks increase or decrease?

The S-REF model further elaborated

In the article "Breaking the Cybernetic Code: Understanding and treating the human metacognitive control system to enhance mental health", Wells (2019) further refines and elaborates on the S-REF model. The purpose of refining the model in this way is to stimulate further research in terms of metacognition, cognitive regulation and effective treatment, based on the current state of knowledge in neuropsychology and metacognition.

The metacognitive control system, the cognitive system and the cybernetic code

In the refined S-REF model, the cognitive and metacognitive systems are further and more clearly separated. A metacognitive control system (MCS) is described, which monitors and controls the activity of the cognitive system (CS) and regulates the activity of neural networks, which in turn affect and affects the ways in which cognition is perceived. The activity in the neural networks can be such as sensory information, gut feeling, arousal, salience, reward, etcetera.

The metacognitive control system consists of a comparative mechanism and metacognitive knowledge in the form of declarative and procedural knowledge and a cybernetic code. The declarative knowledge, "d-knowledge", in the metacognitive control system, is described as a library of data about thinking, stored in long-term memory to be used for self-regulation. The d-knowledge in MCS is often represented as metacognitive beliefs such as "Some thoughts are dangerous" or "It's important to worry about everything that can go wrong". D-knowledge is thus involved in the monitoring and processing of data from the cognitive and metacognitive systems.

The procedural knowledge, the "p-knowledge", in the metacognitive control system is used to regulate by providing instructions or programs to control metacognitive and cognitive activity when cognitive errors or discrepancies according to metacognitive goals have been noted. An example of a p-knowledge-initiated instruction could be: "Continue to ruminate on why you don't feel happy!" Temporary memory registers are also assumed to exist. The function of the metacognitive control system is to monitor and control the activities of the cognitive system based on metacognitive goals. The refined S-REF model assumes that the comparative mechanism of the metacognitive control system monitors ongoing cognitive activity and compares this against an internal model. This internal model constitutes a standard for the current and expected state of cognition. In the event of discrepancies between the internal model and ongoing cognitive activity, and when errors are detected, instructions are given via control mechanisms to restore the activity of the cognitive system according to the metacognitive objectives. To enable this control function, the metacognitive control system is assumed to use a cybernetic code that governs and regulates continued cognitive activity.

Worry, rumination, appraisal and behaviors constitute metacognitive strategies but are all processes within the cognitive system. Control, executive processes, metacognitive knowledge, and information about current activity in the cognitive system belongs to the metacognitive control system. In the case of psychological and emotional problems, it is mainly the metacognitive control system that causes bias that can be observed in the cognitive system. From this further development of the S-REF model, it follows even more clearly that the treatment should focus on the identification and modification of metacognitive knowledge, metacognitive strategies and the regulation of the metacognitive control system. Intense CAS in the form of worry and rumination needs to be reduced early in the treatment to enable sufficient space for thought, a space needed to carry out modification of the metacognitive control system. The techniques and dialogues in MCT are designed to keep the therapeutic dialogue in metacognitive mode, which is necessary to modify both declarative and procedural metacognitive knowledge.

The validity of metacognitive beliefs, but not of cognition, is challenged in MCT. Good metacognitive therapy, according to the model, is also one that modifies the procedural knowledge base. The treatment should help the client to be able to change their relationship with the cognitive products (for example, in the face of the thought/product "I am psychologically damaged"). The treatment should also help the client to directly manipulate control over cognition, such as postponing worry or inhibiting perseverative negative thinking. In addition, the treatment should help the client to separate metacognitive control from internal events in the form of feelings and thoughts as well as external events. Through attention exercises, which are carried out within the framework of the metacognitive exploratory dialogue in MCT, the client is given the opportunity to discover that attention remains flexible and that it can be controlled independently of internal and external events.

Emotions in metacognitive therapy

Dysfunctional metacognition has been found to be associated with emotion dysregulation in both nonclinical and clinical populations (Mansueto et al., 2024). MCT is about self-regulation. The goal is to increase the experience of emotional, cognitive and behavioral regulation, but the interventions in MCT are aimed at the regulation of cognition and not directly at the regulation of emotions and behaviors. Clients often seek help with problems with persistent anxiety, fear, sadness and depression. Sometimes one seeks help with anger problems, at other times for problems with jealousy. Many people seek help with stress related problems. Some clients may express that they are unable to initiate or complete important daily routines if they feel bored, distracted or unmotivated. MCT begins with the therapist and client jointly examining the symptoms that the client is bothered by and the emotional problems that are in focus. Despite this, interventions in MCT are not used to directly manage, further nuance or regulate emotions. In MCT, for example, standard CBT techniques are not used to deal with emotions, such as psychoeducation about emotions/affects, applied relaxation, different breathing techniques, acceptance or self-compassion. Nor are cognitive so-called restructuring techniques used to change an emotion by changing the thought content associated with the emotion. The message delivered in MCT is rather: You don't need to control your emotions, let them instead take care of themselves.

According to MCT, problems with the regulation of negative emotions are related to certain thoughts about emotions and to CAS activity related to the emotions. For example, as a client, you may have a belief that certain levels of anxiety are harmful or "too much". When anxiety is phrased as something painful, difficult or very unpleasant, the implicit experience is usually *worry* about what might happen if the anxiety continues or intensifies. In some anxiety problems, it's often obvious that the client experiences the thoughts as more significant when they are concomitant with anxiety. This type of notion can be challenged in MCT with, for example, the question: Does the thought that the plane could crash become more significant if it is associated with anxiety? What would happen if you instead chose to relate to those thoughts and emotions as if they were unimportant? Other examples can be feelings of shame that are dealt with by either submissive behavior or with aggressive, excessively assertive behavior. A closer examination of such reactions could indicate that shame is associated with trigger thoughts about humiliation and inferiority or that trigger thoughts such as "they will laugh at me" or "they don't take me seriously" could be identified. Further examples can be anger and a person who behaves in ways that appear unregulated and frightening to those around him. That person might say something like "When I get angry, I totally lose control over my behavior and no longer know what I'm doing". Thoughts about anger, about impulses in anger and perceptions of loss of control over behavior at a certain intensity of anger could be explored in MCT. Likewise, a dialogue could be initiated about outbursts of anger as a coping strategy in relation to trigger thoughts.

If the client thinks that internal events such as intense emotions and certain thoughts need to be controlled, such beliefs are explored and challenged. When asked about trigger thoughts, the client may object: "I don't think anything special, but my anxiety is so terribly difficult and severe!" In a continued exploratory dialogue, the discovery is usually that what is experienced as difficult is the worry process and the other CAS activity around the anxiety/physiological sensations. Persistent anxiety, depression or stress are a consequence of CAS. The goal of MCT is therefore to systematically address the causes of the difficulties regulating emotion, i.e. reduce CAS. Without ongoing CAS, the emotions will become self-regulating according to the S-REF model. Emotions, such as fear, sadness, anger, or shame, can be understood as basic internal signals of discrepancies in self-regulation and of threats to well-being. Normally, different emotions are of limited duration when the individual engages in coping that reduces the discrepancy in self-regulation. Perhaps irritation is aroused by something the husband has done or not done at home, which gives the person further input to try to discuss the situation with him and thus the matter is acted out? At the very best, that is. On many occasions the coping strategy may be to let the event pass and not engage in the trigger thoughts. In either case, the irritation can be temporary rather than persistent. In clinical practice, the difference between emotion and cognition is not decisive. When the client describes a problematic emotional experience, it means that they are aware of the emotion and thus have thoughts about it. These thoughts about emotion, the physiological sensations, are explored in terms of trigger thoughts, CAS and metacognition. Nor does the difference between emotion and cognition seem to be decisive theoretically. In newer research-based emotion models, previously influential theories about universal and innate basic emotions/emotion categories are refuted; see for example Barrett (2017). Previous divisions between emotion and cognition tend to dissolve, and emotion is described by Barrett not as a reactive process, but as a predictive one. Barrett describes emotions as predictions made based on interoceptive data, external events, life history, and cultural context.

The S-REF model exemplified

The psychologist Maja from Chapter 1, who previously felt lost about how she should be able to choose in an evidence-based way between different diagnosis-specific treatment protocols in comorbid problems, tried this time, after some MCT training, to generate a case formulation based on the S-REF model. Maja's intended client Eva is troubled by alcohol problems, is depressed, faces problems in her relationship and suffers anxiety, stress and worry. In addition, Eva has difficulty sleeping at night and is bothered by obsessive thoughts and compulsions about the stove and other electrical appliances not being turned off. Maja is trained in several diagnosis-specific CBT treatments, but this time it made more sense to choose a transdiagnostic model such as MCT for analysis and treatment.

Maja has conducted the case formulation interview with Eva within the framework of an exploratory metacognitive dialogue. Maja started by asking Eva to describe her symptoms because it is usually natural to start exploring there. When the S-REF model is used as a transdiagnostic case formulation interview, symptoms, physiological sensations and emotions are identified within level 3 (*low-level processing*). Maja placed the symptoms in box level 3, low-level processing. Then Maja and Eva tried to identify a trigger thought from a current situation where Eva had been bothered by the symptoms at level 2. Maja's interview continued when she and Eva together examined how Eva responded to the trigger thought by worry, rumination, threat monitoring and thought control strategies/behaviors. Eva described how she worries that her symptoms will worsen, about her alcohol consumption, that her stress problems will mean that she will never return to work, and that her relationship problems will lead to divorce. Eva often monitors her experience of stress and exhaustion. She ruminates about the reasons why she feels so bad. Eva increasingly avoids engaging in social events outside the home and she uses alcohol to try to reduce stress, anxiety and worry. Maja and Eva then continued to identify positive and negative metacognitive beliefs about CAS at level 1. The generated case formulation is shown in Figure 2.2.

| Level 1: | **Positive metacognitive beliefs**
Rumination helps me understand my problems.
Worry helps me be prepared. |
| | **Negative metacognitive beliefs**
I can't stop worrying, it's uncontrollable
I'll get sick from all the thinking |

Monitoring ↑   ↓ Control

| Level 2: | **Trigger thoughts**
Another meaningless day ahead. Will I ever get well? Did I turn off the stove? What if my husband meets someone else and wants a divorce?

CAS
Worry: What if my health condition worsens?
Rumination: When did everything start to go wrong with me?
Threat monitoring: Of emotions, physiology. How am I feeling?
Behavior: Alcohol, avoiding friends, checking the stove |

Intrusion ↑   ↓ Bias

| Level 3: | **Symptoms / physiology**
Lacking energy, sad, restless, anxious, tense, irritable, obsessive thoughts, sleep problems, easily stressed |

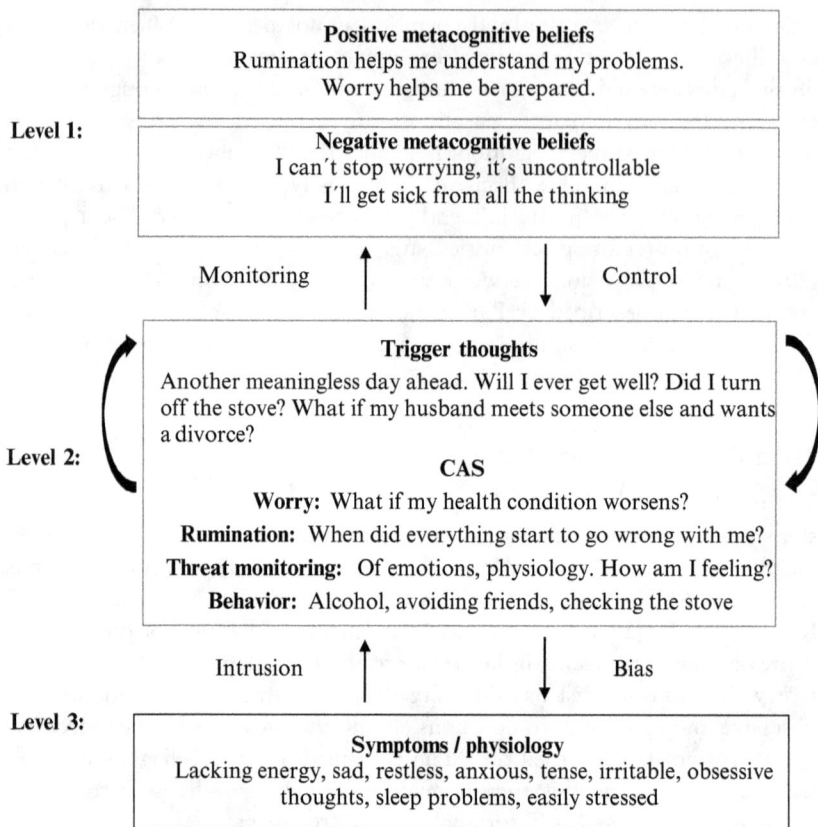

Figure 2.2 The S-REF model, simplified and adapted version, own example comorbid problems, from *Attention and Emotion: A Clinical Perspective*, by Wells and Matthews © (1994) published by Imprint. Reproduced by permission of the Taylor & Francis Group.

In Chapter 9, the reasons for defining MCT as an independent psychotherapy model will be further elaborated. Some techniques and concepts from MCT may seem familiar to clinicians who work within a CBT tradition or within other psychotherapy models. For example, a central intervention in MCT, *detached mindfulness* (DM), may at first glance remind of Buddhist-inspired mindfulness. How DM differs in crucial ways from mindfulness and how techniques in MCT differ from those in other psychotherapy models, is described further in Chapter 4.

3   The treatment, Part I

Overview of the treatment

The treatment is theory-driven

It may be worth reminding the reader that MCT is not about the therapist delivering a set of therapeutic techniques or modules. In fact, a skilled therapist needs to use relatively few techniques to bring about significant metacognitive change and symptom reduction. The treatment is not technique-driven. Instead, MCT is a clearly theory-driven treatment designed to target and change the causal mechanisms behind the client's symptoms. The interventions are thus not directly aimed at reducing symptoms such as anxiety, but at the mechanisms that cause and maintain the symptoms, which according to the model is CAS and dysfunctional metacognition.

In the chapter, there are vignettes with imaginary dialogues between the therapist (T) and the client (P) to illustrate what the interventions, within the framework of the metacognitive dialogue, can look like. These dialogues are fictitious. For even more detailed descriptions, structured interview protocols and for special treatment protocols for generalized anxiety disorder (GAD), post-traumatic stress disorder (PTSD), obsessive-compulsive disorder (OCD) and major depression, see Wells (2009).

Principles and interventions

Emotional and psychological problems are explained by the CAS and by dysfunctional metacognition, according to MCT. The overall goal of the treatment is thus to modify the metacognitive beliefs that have previously caused CAS and to eliminate or reduce CAS. This overall goal also includes increasing executive control of attention so that attention can be used more flexibly, as well as increasing behaviors that promote vitality and well-being. One of the central interventions to reduce CAS is *detached mindfulness* (DM). DM is about noting a thought as separate from the self and refraining from further response to or involvement in the thought. Since CAS implies responding to the trigger, DM is the antithesis of CAS. In Chapter 4, detached mindfulness is described in more detail under a specific heading. Special techniques aimed to increase flexible control of attention, exercises

DOI: 10.4324/9781003597100-4

which will later be described in that chapter, are also important interventions to achieve the treatment goals.

On theoretical and methodological integrity in MCT

MCT is a qualified theory-driven treatment and should not be mixed with other forms of psychotherapy. Eclectically incorporating new techniques from different theoretical models is a common procedure in contemporary psychotherapy approaches, but it does not work in MCT; the treatment would then lose its rigor, quality and its distinct direction. One of the strengths of MCT is that the treatment emanates from the empirically based theoretical model and from the case formulation, and that the message is logically very consistent: The problems arise and persist when you engage in negative thoughts repetitively. As well as responding to your thoughts, you will find that it is possible and safe to leave them alone, whenever you wish.

Therapeutic messages about the importance of processing, for example, emotional problems or traumatic memories become contradictory with detached mindfulness (DM) and with the principle of letting cognitions and emotions regulate themselves. Interventions aimed at "processing" instead risk leading to increased rumination and worry and to continued engagement in negative thoughts and memories. The objection from the MCT therapist could be: What is the goal if you want to process emotions or memories? If the goal is to be able to free yourself from painful thoughts and memories, to be able to leave them behind, how about exploring whether that goal can be achieved effectively in more immediate and direct ways?

Several therapeutic interventions from other psychotherapy approaches, such as applied relaxation, breathing techniques, various emotion regulation techniques, self-compassion, acceptance, Buddhist-inspired mindfulness and cognitive restructuring, become incompatible with MCT. For example, questioning or restructuring negative thoughts or schemas becomes theoretically contradictory to the S-REF model. According to S-REF, the content of trigger thoughts don't matter, and what in cognitive therapy is labeled as "schemas" or "core beliefs" are not understood as the cause of mental illness but instead as additional thoughts and as products and consequences of the CAS. Traditional skills training is not used in MCT. Problems are not understood as skill deficiencies, but as negative consequences of CAS. That is, because of worry and rumination, the client often develops *thoughts* (which were discussed in Chapter 2) about their own skill deficiencies. According to MCT, dealing with negative thoughts with *compassion* is to respond to thoughts instead of leaving them behind. Buddhist-inspired mindfulness risks encouraging more thought processing and more self-focused attention. In addition, Buddhist-inspired mindfulness is not a clearly defined psychological concept and by that far less accurate than the concept of detached mindfulness. "Acceptance" becomes a superfluous theoretical concept from the point of the S-REF model and does not add anything important or new, and acceptance-oriented interventions risk stimulating overthinking. Questions that can be raised about acceptance from the MCT perspective are What does it really mean to accept? To accept a thought, is it to do nothing with it or is it to do something? A central principle of MCT is cognitive flexibility, i.e. the experience of freedom of choice between responding to a thought or not.

Different techniques from other psychotherapy approaches, designed to reduce anxiety, also become incompatible with the S-REF model. According to MCT, the interventions should instead be directed at the processes that cause anxiety and emotion regulation difficulties, i.e. directly at CAS and at the meta-beliefs that control the CAS. Similarly, exposure according to the habituation rationale or inhibitory learning rationale (Craske et al., 2014) becomes incompatible with MCT. Such interventions stimulate a continued dialogue at the object level rather than at the metacognitive level and risk being intertwined with messages that anxiety and trigger thoughts are important internal events. In MCT, the message is the opposite, and the client is encouraged to reduce the focus on anxiety and trigger thoughts and instead relate to them as temporary inner events that come and go. In cases where the client describes problems with anxiety, it is possible to identify and intervene against worry and other CAS around the physiological anxiety sensation.

To conduct the treatment with the intended high quality and adherence to the method, the therapist must have completed formal training and supervision in MCT and allow the interventions to be guided logically from the S-REF model and case formulation.

Necessary competence of the therapist

MCT is an advanced evidence-based treatment. Of course, it is essential that the psychologist/psychotherapist has completed proper training and supervision in MCT.[1] The therapist needs to have a well-integrated theoretical and clinical understanding of the theoretical model, the treatment principles, and the therapeutic techniques. The interventions in MCT follow logically and consistently from the theoretical model and the individual case formulation. The therapist needs to be able to detect and make the client aware of when the CAS is activated, what trigger thoughts preceded the activation of CAS and which meta-beliefs currently control the CAS. Another prerequisite for the therapy to be carried out with the intended quality, is that the therapist recognizes and can easily differentiate between object mode and metacognitive mode dialogues. The therapist needs to be able to switch the dialogue from the object level to the metacognitive level and to hold the dialogue there. It is very easy to linger and get stuck in dialogues at the level of thought content in clinical conversations, but such dialogues do not become therapeutically effective according to MCT. Examples of object-level questions could be: "Will I ever be able to feel happy again?" or "Am I starting to become more and more like my father who was also depressed?"

A continued dialogue at the object level rather stimulates continued or increased rumination and worry. When this happens, the dialogue needs to be switched to metacognitive mode, to a dialogue about thoughts, such as "How are you affected emotionally when you think about it?" or "If you find that those thoughts don't lead you forward, can you leave them alone?". Clinicians who are lacking proper and appropriate training in MCT will also be tempted to compensate for insufficient competence by also incorporating analysis models and treatment interventions from other psychotherapy models. The therapeutic procedure then becomes eclectic, imprecise/confusing and will also be delivered from an unknown state of empirical evidence.

The interaction between therapist and client should be a joint explorative dialogue. The therapist asks metacognitive questions that will facilitate the client's discoveries about their own thinking and about how cognition and emotions can be regulated in more helpful and effective ways. In addition to being explorative, the dialogue is designed to challenge, test and modify dysfunctional metacognitive beliefs. The verbal and behavioral challenge of metacognitive beliefs should always be done with a friendly, genuinely empathetic and interested exploratory attitude from the therapist. Debate, persuasion, or irony have of course no place here. The interventions, when skillfully implemented, should both increase the patient's curiosity about their own mental model, about problematic thought processes and meta-beliefs, as well as their motivation to experiment with new and more helpful strategies, strategies that will enable the modification of previous dysfunctional metacognition. A clinician without sufficient training and supervision in the method will have difficulty conducting and maintaining an effective metacognitive dialogue.

Overview, structure of the treatment course and of the treatment session

MCT is usually a short-term therapy. Treatment protocols for GAD, PTSD, OCD, and depression (Wells, 2009) range in length from 8 up to 10 sessions. An experienced and well-trained therapist can often complete the therapy with achieved treatment goals faster than that. The treatment is sequential, and the interventions targeted at dysfunctional metacognition and the CAS take place in a specific order. Even if the treatment protocol for GAD, for example, specifies what should be done session by session, the therapist does usually not proceed in the protocol until, for example, negative meta-beliefs about uncontrollability have been significantly reduced. Thus, depending on how the treatment process has progressed, working with, for example, session 5 according to the protocol, could in practice mean that it is the client's and therapist's fourth or sixth session in the therapy process. Normally, the work is first focused on reducing worry and/or rumination and somewhat later in the treatment on reducing CAS behaviors. When the problems are severe, for example, when personality disorders are part of the clinical picture, the treatment is often longer than 8–10 sessions. For example, in the treatment of borderline personality disorder, the treatment, together with other interventions, has been time-bound up to one year (Nordahl & Wells, 2019).

MCT always begins with a case formulation interview to identify triggers, and explore the client's CAS profile, how symptoms are maintained through CAS, and metacognitive beliefs. The client is then socialized to the model, a dialogue which aims to increase their awareness of how the case formulation and the model explain the symptoms and problems. During the socialization the therapist checks if the case formulation makes sense to the patient and whether it fits with the patient's experience of their psychological problems. When it is evident to the therapist and client that the CAS and metacognitive beliefs explain the maintenance of the problems, the bridge to the treatment is introduced. The bridging means that, in the light of the case formulation, the therapist briefly conveys alternative ways of relating to triggers, alternative attention strategies and alternative metacognitive beliefs and plans.

Negative metacognitive beliefs about worry and rumination as uncontrollable and dangerous thought processes and about trigger thoughts as powerful and dangerous, are considered more important for symptom development and maintenance and thus more prioritized to start modifying than the positive meta-beliefs. Prolonged worry and rumination bring so many negative consequences that these components of CAS become important to reduce as soon as possible. Worry and rumination occupy much of the cognitive resources that need to be freed up for change to take place. To reduce and interrupt worry, the client is introduced to the alternative of *detached mindfulness* (DM), i.e. "non-response", meaning that for the moment there should be no response at all to the trigger thought. In addition, experiments with postponement of worry/rumination are introduced as a new strategy. The client is then encouraged to postpone worry or rumination until a short moment of thinking towards the end of the day. According to the experiment, whether the time for thinking should be used later is voluntary. In depressive rumination and in the case of social anxiety, attention exercises are introduced, which aim among other things to interrupt rumination and threat monitoring, increase the perception of control of thought processes and employ a more flexible use of attention.

Verbal and behavioral techniques to further reduce worry, rumination and other CAS, as well as to modify metacognitive beliefs, are used throughout the course of therapy. Detached mindfulness, different attention exercises, postponement of worry/rumination and reduction of avoidance, threat monitoring, and other CAS, are also given as homework assignments between therapy sessions. One overall goal is that the client should develop new strategies that are to be generalized, used in life outside the therapist's office and with the ability to function in the long term. The treatment process is continuously monitored with special rating scales for assessment of CAS and metacognition, ratings that also guide the therapist in the choice of further interventions. When it comes to modifying metacognitive beliefs, the approach is that negative meta-beliefs about uncontrollability are usually prioritized first, then negative beliefs about worry/rumination as dangerous processes, and finally positive meta-beliefs. In some cases, positive metacognitive beliefs, or fusion beliefs, can block further interventions aiming at reducing worry/rumination, for example if the client does not dare to reduce worry or seems very hesitant to reduce rumination. Different forms of blocking beliefs then need to be identified and modified before further work can be done to reduce worry/rumination and negative meta-beliefs. Prior to the termination of the treatment, important discoveries made during treatment, new metacognitive knowledge that the client has acquired and will be able to use in the future, are summarized. The therapist and the client draw up a new plan together for how the updated metacognitive knowledge and strategies can be maintained in the long term.

The metacognitive dialogue permeates all MCT. Instead of giving the client psychoeducation or advice in the form of didactic instructions, the dialogue is characterized by guided and joint exploration. It is not possible to teach someone to ride a bike by giving explanations, and similarly, metacognitive change is an experiential process. The form of dialogue is often perceived as new and unfamiliar. Most of us are not used to identifying what type of trigger thought we have in a situation of stress or negative affect, how we then relate to such a thought or what ideas we then have about worry or rumination as thought processes. To stop and reflect on questions about how we come to make certain thoughts more important than others, and what consequences this has for us, usually feels unfamiliar. Nor are we usually used to considering the problems in our lives based on a metacognitive explorative dialogue about how often we think about the problem, how we feel when we think about it persistently, and whether this form of thinking leads us forward or rather makes us feel paralyzed and confused. Spontaneously, many clients express after the first or second MCT session and when socializing to the model and case formulation: "This is exactly how it goes and how I think and function. I do recognize myself in the model". Similar reactions are of course signs that the client feels that the symptoms and problems can be better explained by the S-REF model than by external events, life history or biological processes.

Unhelpful, or even counterproductive behaviors, such as avoidance or substance use/abuse can usually be understood as secondary CAS, i.e. as secondary strategies, aimed at reducing worry and rumination. CAS behaviors thus become much easier to reduce somewhat later, when worry and rumination have decreased, when uncontrollability beliefs have been reduced and when the client has discovered alternative and more effective ways to interrupt worry and rumination. In cases where the client's behaviors become directly dangerous or impede continued therapy, these need to be addressed and prioritized. Examples of such problematic behaviors can be self-harm, substance abuse or a lack of routines for eating and sleeping. In cases where there is a significant acute risk of suicidal acts, this risk should be managed according to current clinical guidelines in psychiatric care. Otherwise, the starting point is that destructive or self-sabotaging behaviors can also be understood according to the S-REF model and based on the case formulation. Here, the therapist and the client need to come to a common understanding of the function of the behavior according to S-REF and to a common goal and plan on how the behavior can be reduced. In cases where highly self-destructive behaviors occur, the therapist needs to make it clear that the common goal naturally needs to be about removing the obstacles that exist to the improved health and improved mental well-being of the client.

At the beginning of the treatment, the focus is on reducing worry and rumination and on modifying metacognitive beliefs about uncontrollability. In depressive states, characterized by intense rumination and self-focused attention, or in social anxiety, a lot of focus is initially on behavioral experiments, on how attention can be varied and manipulated. The rationale for these exercises is, among other things, that the client should be able to experience how the focus of attention affects the symptoms, and that attention is under executive control. Through exercises where the client increases the external focus of attention, it becomes easier to interrupt rumination and to engage in social conversations and interaction.

As worry and rumination have decreased and the client's experience of being able to control these thought processes has increased, metacognitive beliefs about the dangers of these thought processes have often already diminished. Worry and rumination that can be interrupted at any time are rarely perceived as dangerous in the same way as before. Anyone who believes that worry is harmful could now choose to interrupt the worry process instead of continuing. When uncontrollability beliefs have been radically reduced, remaining danger meta-beliefs are explored, challenged and modified with verbal techniques and with behavioral experiments. After the uncontrollability beliefs have been modified, the treatment interventions are also directed towards the cessation of avoidance and other CAS behaviors. As mentioned earlier, it will now be much easier for the client to feel confident that worry and rumination can be controlled in other ways than by, for example, avoidance, alcohol/substances or by asking relatives or friends for reassurance.

Towards the end of the treatment the therapeutic interventions are systematically focused on modifying remaining positive meta-beliefs about the CAS. Finally, the therapist and client establish a new plan, a maintenance plan, which describes how the client will continue to use the new strategies that have been practiced in therapy, in terms of detached mindfulness, postponement of worry/rumination, external and flexible use of attention and increased activities. Considering that worry and rumination have indeed been very resource demanding, tiring and draining processes, there is usually a very good prospect that the client will find it easier and more appealing in the long term to stick to the new plan than to return to the old one, i.e. the CAS. Why return to something that is unnecessarily energy-consuming and that causes emotional dysregulation?

The interventions to reduce CAS and modify meta-beliefs are thus based both on verbal exploratory dialogues and on experience-based exercises and experiments. The following describes in more detail different sequences of treatment and interventions used.

Typically, treatment sessions last for about 45–50 minutes and are scheduled weekly, at least initially during treatment and until significant progress has been made. There are some similarities with CBT, but also crucial differences. Several of the elements that are emphasized in CBT regarding the session structure and core therapeutic skills, are also emphasized in MCT. In some of the most widely used scales of therapeutic competence in CBT, such as CTRS (Young & Beck, 1980) or CTS-R (Blackburn et al., 2001), several competencies are defined that should be clearly observable and included during the treatment session. Some items that are considered as core competencies according to CTRS and CTS-R regarding the structure of the treatment hour, are also central in MCT. MCT also emphasizes that the treatment sessions should be focused and clearly structured around the overall goal. In MCT, however, this goal is about reducing CAS and dysfunctional metacognition. In MCT, too, the sessions begin with agenda-setting. The therapist has suggestions about the agenda informed by the treatment model, based on the phase of the treatment one is in and based on the CAS and the meta-beliefs that still exist. The client is encouraged to participate actively and provide input based on their own experience regarding the agenda, the interventions, and the treatment process. If deviations are made from the established agenda, this should be done in a transparent manner and be justified based on the treatment goals. During the session, recurring summaries are made where the therapist asks for feedback and gives feedback. The therapy session should be characterized by active collaboration between client and therapist and the therapeutic dialogue by guided exploration (but in MCT it is about guided exploration at the metacognitive level). Therapist and client explore together how the client's thought processes affect symptoms and emotional well-being, and how certain behavioral strategies exacerbate symptoms and can lead to emotional dysregulation, and how alternative behaviors contribute to recovery. New homework assignments are formulated based on the theme that has been relevant during the session, and these are followed up at the next session. Contrary to what is expected in CBT with, for example, CTRS or CTS-R, during the MCT session there is of course no exploration, questioning or restructuring of thought content or of schema. During the MCT session, it is emphasized that the dialogue should mostly take place on the metacognitive level and that the therapist shows competence in switching up the dialogue from the object level to the metacognitive level.

Continuous measurements of CAS and metacognition

Given that the goal is to reduce or eliminate CAS and dysfunctional metacognition, continuous measurements and continuous feedback are needed to monitor and ensure that this is really happening. CAS and metacognition are to be understood as interacting systems. This means that interventions aimed at reducing CAS also affect metacognition and vice versa. CAS and metacognitive beliefs are continuously measured each session using special rating scales, of which the psychometric properties are largely unexplored (Wells, 2009). In the treatment of GAD, the scale GADS-R is used, in the treatment of PTSD the scale PTSD-S, in OCD the scale OCD-S and in the treatment of depression the MDD-S. In these scales, worry, rumination, threat monitoring and behavior/avoidance are measured on a Likert scale from 0 to 8. Dysfunctional metacognitive beliefs are measured on scales between 0 and 100. Metacognitive measurements such as "how much do you think your worry is uncontrollable on a scale from 0 to 100?" as well as levels of worry, rumination and other CAS, help the therapist to monitor the treatment process and to systematically choose further interventions. A generic CAS-1 rating scale has also been developed for the same purpose as the scales above. CAS-1 can be chosen when treatment is focused on comorbid problems.

At the beginning of the treatment, the therapist follows up by ascertaining that worry and rumination decrease as intended, then that CAS behaviors and avoidance are decreasing. In the beginning, there are also negative meta-beliefs about uncontrollability that the therapist needs to follow up to ensure that these are reduced. Prior to the end of treatment, the goal is for the ratings of CAS and meta-beliefs to be close to 0. In addition to the use of rating scales before each session, verbal ratings of the current metacognitive belief are also asked for before and after a chosen intervention. If the goal with a chosen intervention is to reduce the meta-belief that worry is uncontrollable, the therapist asks for both pre- and post-ratings of the belief on a scale between 0 and 100. If the client has had some success in reducing the worry by postponing it (see further in Chapter 4 on postponement of worry and rumination), the therapist asks for a new rating of the uncontrollability belief, which would then be expected to have decreased.

Treatment format

The most common and most tested treatment protocols (Wells, 2009) describe MCT in an individual format. Based on preliminary studies, MCT also seems to be an effective group treatment (Callesen et al., 2019; Dammen et al., 2015, 2016; Hammersmark et al., 2024; Haseth et al., 2019; Papageorgiou et al., 2018; Wells et al., 2021). An advantage of MCT in a group setting can be that clients in one sense feel that they have individual problems that can be experienced as unique and private, but in another sense, they know that everyone else in the group also has problems with worry and rumination and that the content of the thoughts does not matter. MCT has also been studied in a self-help format with cardiovascular patients with anxiety and depression problems, and shown to be an effective (Wells et al., 2023) and meaningful intervention (Wells et al., 2022b).

Metacognitive case formulation and socialization

As mentioned earlier, metacognitive therapy always begins with case formulation. This means that the client describes their problems and that the client and therapist then together map the symptoms, trigger thoughts, the CAS profile and the metacognitive beliefs that are controlling the CAS. The case formulation is carried out in the form of a structured interview with questions in a predetermined logical order. For example, if worry is included as a significant symptom-generating process, different worry themes are mapped, as well as how long and at what moments the client worries. In addition, the negative consequences that result from worry in terms of anxiety, stress, fatigue, concentration problems, impaired self-esteem and strained interpersonal relationships with, for example, partner and family, are explored. The client's attempts to reduce worry with, for example, thought suppression, distraction or other strategies are identified and discussed. Similarly, if rumination occurs, questions are asked about how often and for how long the client ruminates over different themes, as well as about the negative consequences of rumination. Any internal monitoring of emotions, physiology, or motivation is mapped as well as external threat monitoring being identified. It is likely that the client discovers already during the case formulation that their coping strategies work poorly and that they even have a paradoxical effect on perceived stress. Here it becomes obvious to both client and therapist that ineffective coping strategies increase the experience of worry and rumination as uncontrollable and even harmful processes. Positive and negative meta-beliefs about worry/rumination are identified and discussed. Does the client believe that the worry is necessary and helpful, perhaps even vital, while at the same time finding it deeply disturbing and problematic? Does the client believe that worry is uncontrollable and dangerous?

In some conditions, the client's metacognitive awareness tends to be low. If, for example, a depressed client initially does not recognize that he or she ruminates to any great extent, the case formulation also aims to explore more closely the very existence of rumination, to raise awareness that this thought process is nevertheless active to a significant extent, and to map how rumination affects the mood negatively. Furthermore, the case formulation and subsequent socialization can aim to clarify that the client's problem is to be understood as a metacognitive problem. An example here could be an OCD client with extensive contamination fear. Through the formulation of the case and subsequent socialization, the conditions are created for the client to realize more fundamentally that their problems are not about hygiene and dirt, but about thoughts and thinking about all of this.

Socialization means that the therapist and the client create a common understanding of the processes that cause and maintain the symptoms and problems based on the case formulation. Socialization is also carried out within the framework of an explorative dialogue in which several negative consequences are clarified. What are the consequences for the client if they are convinced that worry is both something harmful to their health and at the same time something vital to reduce the risk of illness and accidents? What are the consequences for emotional regulation and self-image of believing that worry is uncontrollable? How does such a meta-belief affect any attempt to discontinue worry or rumination? Through socialization, the negative consequences of believing that the worry is harmful can also be clarified. Furthermore, socialization can clarify the consequences of fusion meta-beliefs when they occur. What are the consequences of believing that certain thoughts are dangerous and could have the power to get the client to act in a way that they do not want to?

Furthermore, through socialization, a bridge to treatment takes place by the therapist asking explorative hypothetical questions about what a life without CAS and without dysfunctional metacognition could look like. An example of such a bridging question could be: "If you discovered that you could choose to refrain from ruminating whenever you wish, what would that mean for you?" In connection with socialization, a plan is introduced for how CAS can be reduced, and how metacognitive beliefs can be tested and challenged.

Special case-formulation interviews are included in the specific treatment protocols designed for the treatment of generalized anxiety disorder (GAD), post-traumatic stress disorder (PTSD), obsessive-compulsive disorder (OCD), and depression, and these are found in Wells (2009).

The AMC model

A generic case formulation can also be made according to the AMC model, where A stands for internal **antecedent**, M for **metacognitive beliefs** and CAS, and C for emotional **consequences** (Wells, 2000, 2009). AMC is a reformulated ABC model, which is an analysis model used in CBT where A stands for antecedent/trigger, B for **beliefs** (i.e. dysfunctional core beliefs or schemas) and C stands for **consequences**, emotional and behavioral (i.e. consequences of core beliefs for emotion and behavior). Since core beliefs/schemas have no explanatory value in the S-REF model, B is replaced by M in AMC. In addition, the antecedent in AMC becomes a trigger thought, unlike ABC analysis, where A can stand for a situation where the symptoms were activated.

The AMC model can be understood as a variant of the S-REF model, but graphically the model is set up horizontally, rather than vertically as with the S-REF. The interview is usually conducted "backwards" in the sense that the therapist starts by asking questions about C, i.e. the emotional symptoms the client has been bothered by during the past two weeks, and then asks questions about A, an activating internal event, i.e. about the trigger linked to a sudden change in emotional state. Finally, M, i.e. meta-cognition and CAS, is explored. The questions are first asked about CAS, i.e. about how the client responded to the trigger in the form of worry, rumination, threat monitoring and behaviors, and then about which metacognitive beliefs were associated with CAS. The AMC interview with a patient with social anxiety could look like this:

T: *Over the past two weeks, what has your social anxiety been like?*
   [Explores C]

P: There have been a couple of difficult situations, but especially one on Thursday last week when I bumped into a very pretty classmate that I had felt a little bit in love with.

T: *What happened then?*

P: I felt completely panicked, stupid and almost couldn't get a word out when she started talking to me.

T: *What do you think was the first thought you had in that situation?*
   [Searching for A]

P: I felt like a mental case. Like an idiot. So, the thought was probably something like "She must think I'm really weird".

T: *When you felt so nervous, blocked, and had that thought, what happened to your thinking? [Exploring M and starting with CAS]*

P: I started to worry about what she really thinks of me and that she would find the situation difficult and unpleasant.

T: *Did anything special happen to your attention?*

P: I became very self-conscious and preoccupied with how stiff and strange I must have looked in her eyes.

T: *Did you in any way try to deal with your emotions or how you may have appeared?*

P: I think I put my hands in my pants pockets to hide that they were shaking, and I probably smiled a lot more than I usually do to try to mask the panic I felt. I started yawning too as an attempt to relax a bit.

T: *Did you try to push away some thoughts?*

P: Somehow everything went so fast, but I think I struggled with trying to get rid of the thought "Now she thinks I'm really strange".

T: *It seems that your worry and attention focus on your symptoms and on your nervous appearance, as you imagined it in the situation, didn't make it any easier for you?*

P: No, it made the situation much worse.

T: *If you were to be asked why you don't stop worrying, what would your answer be? [Examines M further and now a negative meta-belief about uncontrollability]*

P: That's easier said than done. I find it impossible to stop worrying about my stiff and nervous appearance in those situations.

T: *Do you see any benefits in trying to imagine what she thinks of you when you're nervous or what she thinks of you after such situations? [Explores M further and initiates here the mapping of positive meta-beliefs]*

P: I'm not sure about that, but I guess I need to know if she sees me as a pitiful, scared wretch or not ...

A	M	C
Antecedent/ Trigger	**Metacognitive beliefs**	**Emotional and behavioral consequences**
I probably appear like a mental case. She thinks that I'm really weird.	Worry helps me find answers to whether she thinks I´m pitiful and weak. I can´t help but to worry in those situations.	Panicked, blocked, fell silent.

CAS
I worry about what she thinks of me and whether she finds the situation unpleasant
Attention focused on the symptoms and my own nervous appearance.
Behavior/Thought control
Hid shaking hands. Yawned. Tried to suppress negative thoughts

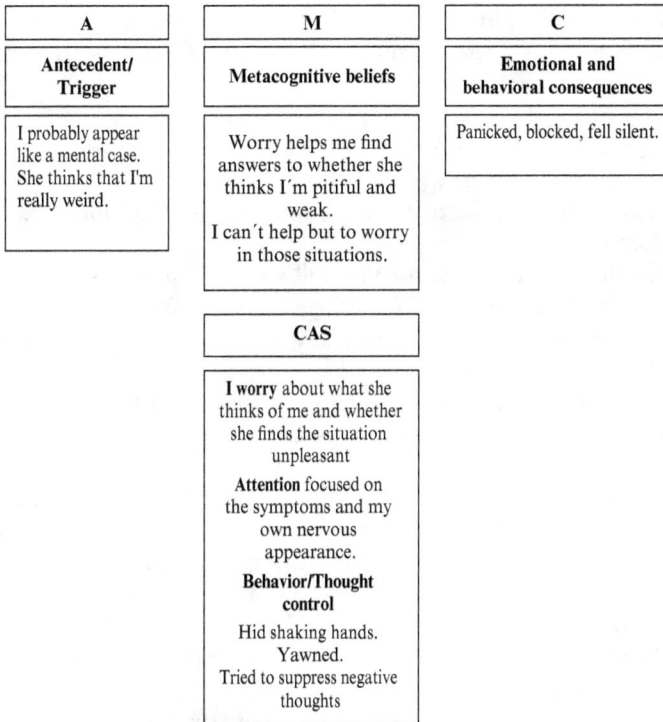

Figure 3.1 AMC formulation in social anxiety. Simplified, redrawn model from Wells (2000, 2009). Own example.

Behavioral assessment tests (BATs)

Some clients may find it difficult answering questions about C, that is, about the emotional symptoms during the AMC interview. It may thus be more difficult to also identify trigger thought, CAS and metacognition according to AMC. These may be clients with a pronounced and long-term avoidance of anxiety-provoking situations and anxious thoughts. The client may find it hard to recall a reasonably current situation that was emotionally charged. In these cases, the AMC interview can be combined with a behavioral assessment test designed to break the avoidance and with the aim that the client will get in touch with the emotional symptoms. For a person with social anxiety and pronounced avoidance, a behavioral assessment test can be suggested, which means that the client is asked to start a conversation with a stranger. Sometimes it may be enough to start with the emotional reaction that the proposal alone evokes in the client. Otherwise, this test is carried out with the AMC interview immediately afterwards. A client with OCD and fear of contamination may be asked to either engage in a conversation about what is typically avoided, such as body excretions, or to touch a surface that is typically perceived as dirty. The AMC interview can then continue, and with a patient with health anxiety, it could look something like this after the behavioral assessment test:

T: *Okay, now you've googled for a while on various symptoms that can occur in ALS. You usually try to avoid thoughts of ALS and other diseases. Would you like to tell me how you feel right now? [Starting to explore C]*

P: It was quite scary, I feel nauseous, dull and a bit shaky.

T: *Okay, scared, nauseous, dull and even shaky. What thoughts popped into your mind when you googled and felt scared? [Continuing with exploring A]*

P: I started to think that I quite often feel nauseous, a bit shaky and weak and if it could be that I suffer from serious health problems, for example from ALS.

T: *When you got the idea that maybe you might be seriously ill after all, what did you do? Did you start worrying? Did you start analyzing/ pondering what could speak for and against you being seriously ill? [Starting to explore CAS under M in AMC]*

P: I began to worry that it could already be too late and that these anxiety problems, as I have understood them to be, rather may be diffuse signs of a neurological disease.

T: *Did anything special happen to your attention? Did you become more aware of your physical symptoms?*

P: Yes, I suddenly became very aware of nausea and other physiological symptoms. I think I started scanning my body for those symptoms.

T: *Did you try control the thoughts of ALS in any way? Did you try to shut them out? [Investigating thought suppression as part of CAS]*

P: Yes, at some point I kind of said to myself: "Now you're there painting hell on the wall again. Sharpen up, don't get into those ALS thoughts!"

T: *Do you see any benefits to worrying about ALS? [Begins to explore metacognitive beliefs, M in AMC]*

P: Not really, but somehow, I still think it's good to try to be aware of symptoms like these in time, so that you can at least plan your life somewhat in the face of serious illness.

T: *If you should instead conclude that the involvement in the thoughts of illness is still mostly a problem for you, do you feel that you can decide not to worry? Do you believe your worry and rumination about ALS is possible to control?*

Therapeutic interventions, verbal and behavioral techniques

As already mentioned, the metacognitive dialogue is fundamental in MCT. The case formulation, the socialization and therapeutic interventions are carried out within this dialogue. To explore, challenge and modify metacognitive beliefs, both verbal and behavioral techniques are needed. In most sessions, the therapist uses a mix of verbal and behavioral techniques. The patient needs to try out and experience new ways to relate to and to regulate cognition, and a therapeutic goal is an updated model of the mind, i.e. updated metacognitive knowledge, both at the declarative and procedural level. The next chapter, Chapter 4, gives further and more detailed examples on various interventions to challenge and modify dysfunctional metacognition.

Switching from object mode to a metacognitive dialogue

In the clinical situation, it is common for the client to initially experience and describe the symptoms from the object mode. That is, the client does not usually say that it is the relationship to thoughts that is the problem. Instead, it may be communicated by the client that negative self-esteem causes the problems, one's own inability, depression, severe anxiety, uncertainty about future career or the risk of accidentally forgetting to lock the front door that pose problems. The client may initially be convinced that it is external factors in the environment that cause psychological problems, either here and now or from previous history when growing up. Or the client may be convinced that it is their own biology or a disturbed brain function that is the root of the problems. The MCT therapist initially works to switch the dialogue about the problem formulation from the object level to a metacognitive level. Regardless of previous negative life experiences, current life situation and the client's imagined individual neurobiological constitution, the starting point and prediction is that, to a very significant degree, the client's problems can be understood and treated in terms of CAS and metacognitive beliefs. This shifting of the dialogue from the object level to the metacognitive level should be done in a friendly and empathetic manner, as guided discovery. The therapist asks questions about trigger thoughts in different problem situations, about the emotions associated with these triggers and about how the client relates to trigger thoughts. Furthermore, the therapist asks questions about when, how often and for how long the client spends time worrying or ruminating. To identify trigger thoughts and how the client responds to these in problem situations is to increase metacognitive awareness. Such a dialogue where the therapist works to move from a dialogue at the object level to a metacognitive dialogue could look like this:

P: I know I've been injured and suffer from brain fatigue after all the stress I experienced last year. I should have been more careful, but I just ignored it. Instead, I had a breakdown and a complete collapse.

T: *Is that something you often think about, that you are damaged by stress?*

P: I know that for sure. My family doctor has also told me so.

T: *Okay I see, but is that also something you often think about?*

P: Yes, I'm thinking about it every day.

T: *For how long can the thinking go on?*

P: Oh, for a very long time. I can get stuck in thoughts like that where I wonder why I wasn't gentler with myself as well as when the first symptoms appeared.

T: *What do you usually come up with when you try to understand such things?*

P: Well, admittedly, ... not much at all. Rather like I get tangled up in thoughts and just feel more stressed and even damaged. Like I can't even use my brain to think with anymore.

Another example of a patient who suffers problems with negative self-view and worries about flaws in appearance could look like this:

P: I feel like I look grotesque. My throat and lips look absolutely disgusting and repel other people.

T: *This sounds difficult for you. How often do you think about your appearance as disgusting and repelling?*

P: It's not something I'm thinking. I know my throat and lips look disgusting.

T: *Okay, but even if you say you know, is it also something that you think about when you are alone or have other people around you?*

P: I'm not sure, but of course I react. I don't want others to feel disgusted when they see me.

T: *It sounds like you worry a lot about that. May I ask you, do you have a problem with others telling you that they feel disgusted by your appearance or rather with worry that they might feel that way?*

Some clients who are bothered by compulsions or various forms of tics or trichotillomania do not indicate any obsessions or catastrophic thoughts that should be neutralized with the behavior or ritual. Instead, the description can be that you perform the action to "feel just right" or in some way "need the action to be complete". A dialogue that aims to increase meta-cognitive awareness and to switch from object mode to metacognitive mode could in such cases look like this:

T: When I asked you what would happen if you didn't straighten the carpet edge in your living room at home so that it is exactly straight or if you didn't arrange the objects on your desk symmetrically, you said that you don't worry about anything special happening. Just that it feels right only when you have arranged it completely symmetrically.

P: Yes, that's right. It just doesn't feel right otherwise, like something isn't complete.

T: *What's the problem for you if it doesn't feel quite right or complete?*

P: I don't know. It's just a feeling I suppose. A kind of discomfort, like an internal itch.

T: *Could the trigger thought in such situations be "right now it really doesn't feel right"?*

P: Well, whether it's a distinct thought, I really don't know, but it's kind of an experience that I want to get rid of and that's when I start arranging things so compulsively.

T: *If you imagine that you didn't respond to that feeling, what do you think would happen?*

P: Ugh, that sounds very unpleasant. Then I wouldn't get rid of the feeling. I would feel restless and nervous. I think I would be irritable and later not be able to relax and sleep.

T: *Would you worry that the feeling would last almost forever?*

P: Yes, definitely.

T: *Do you think you would try to change or control the feeling in any way?*

P: I would most likely pay close attention to it. I would probably also try to get rid of the feeling by, for example, turning on a relaxation app that I use sometimes.

T: So does your ritual of symmetrically arranging the objects become a way to regulate worry and the thoughts that otherwise you won't be able to relax?

The therapist thus needs to be able to both switch up the dialogue from the object level to the metacognitive level and kindly and consistently keep the dialogue there. Often, in clinical conversations, the client tends to "slip down" again and return to object-level descriptions of the problems.

Normalization of thoughts and symptoms

When socializing to the case formulation and prior to continued treatment, experiences, thoughts and symptoms may often need to be normalized. For example, a client with PTSD may need to know that many of the symptoms are very common and completely normal after a traumatic event. A person who is bothered by obsessive thoughts may need to hear that the presence of intrusive and unpleasant thoughts is considered to belong to normal psychology and that most of the population confirms that they have them. A depressed person may need a dialogue about the normality of occasionally feeling low, tired and uninterested. In MCT, the message is: "You don't have to deal with your symptoms or thoughts. Let them take care of themselves."

Metacognitive behavioral experiments

The behavioral experiments in MCT are often carried out based on the P-E-T-S protocol (Wells, 1997, 2009), i.e. on the four components *preparation–exposure–testing–summarizing*. There are behavioral experiments developed to challenge and modify all the types of positive and negative metacognitive beliefs that have been described so far. The first preparatory step (P) is about clarifying the meta-belief to be challenged, evaluating its credibility and formulating an experiment where the belief can be tested. In this step, predictions are also made about what will happen when the belief is tested. The next step (E) is about putting the meta-belief to a test by exposing the client to, for example, an internal event in which the belief is activated, to a certain level of worry or to certain thoughts that are usually avoided. The third step, testing (T), can be to change the behavior during the experiment in a way that challenges the meta-belief. The final step is to summarize (S) what occurred during the experiment and to consider what conclusions can be drawn.

As a matter of fact, in general, many of the interventions in MCT can be defined as experiments, even the entire therapy. The client does not have to believe that the treatment will be helpful from the start. "Would you have anything to lose by trying and seeing what will happen to your worry and to your symptoms?" the therapist may ask a client who initially shows ambivalence. The client can also be informed that the treatment will be evaluated continuously, session by session and jointly by the therapist and client. The important thing is to participate in the therapeutic process, test, take part in the metacognitive dialogue and in various exercises and together with the therapist, continuously evaluate what then happens to the CAS and metacognition. Various DM, worry/rumination, postponement and attention exercises that will be described later in more detail, are usually designed so that you first clarify what you want to test with the exercise, then carry it out, and finally discuss the outcome and conclusions that can be drawn. For example: "Should we try out whether it is possible to do nothing for a moment with a negative thought? What did you discover? Can we try again, but in this way? What happened during the exercise?"

Exposure in metacognitive therapy

Exposure is used as a possible treatment intervention in MCT, but in a different way and with different purposes than in, for example, CBT. Exposure is carried out as a form of behavioral experiment, i.e. according to P-E-T-S. The purpose is not to reduce anxiety or to habituate in the situation, which is otherwise a common purpose in CBT. Nor is the exposure carried out in accordance with an inhibitory learning rationale (Craske et al., 2014). In MCT, significantly shorter and fewer exposures are used than in CBT. What you want to achieve with exposure is to modify metacognitive beliefs. For example, exposure to social anxiety can be done where the client is encouraged to give a short presentation to a group of strangers or to engage in a conversation with a stranger. The purpose of such exposure for a client with social phobia is to be able to discover that even when social anxiety is activated, it is entirely possible to shift the attention away from the emotional experience and from the negative image one has of oneself, i.e. self as social object, and instead direct it towards different people and events in the external environment. That is, conclusions after such exposure can usually be: "It works better for me in a social situation when I turn my attention to the other person I am interacting with. It is neither the internal emotions or thoughts, nor the external events that control my attention. I'm the one who chooses how I use it, no matter what thoughts and emotions I may have". Interoceptive exposure in panic disorder can also be used with a metacognitive rationale. The client can then be asked to induce the physiological sensations that have been perceived as frightening, but with the instructions to refrain from worry and other CAS activity. In this way, a negative belief about the worry as uncontrollable can be challenged and modified (A. Wells, personal communication, November 21, 2022).

In the case of worry problems, the therapist can ask the client to intensify their worry for a while to either challenge meta-beliefs about the worry as uncontrollable or, in another experiment, challenge meta-beliefs about the worry as dangerous and harmful. Both exposure with response prevention (ERP) and exposure with response commission (ERC) occur as treatment interventions.

Exposure in metacognitive therapy is not carried out with the message that the client needs to put up with anxiety or endure it to feel better in the long run. Rather, these are golden opportunities to identify trigger thoughts and explore the CAS in the situation and what happens if the client instead applies DM. Ideas that the client may have that exposure is about "exposing oneself to" or "enduring anxiety" should be met with exploratory questions such as "Exactly what do you think should be endured? What is it that makes this experience aversive or unpleasant?" With similar questions, it becomes possible to identify triggers and CAS according to, for example, the AMC model (previously described in this chapter). Most likely, there will be trigger thoughts about anxiety and worry about worry (type 2 worry) to discover. Clients who try to "endure" during traditional exposure in CBT are likely to engage in various forms of worry and threat monitoring of anxiety/interoceptive data and do not practice DM in these moments. See further on exposure according to ERP and ERC in Chapter 4, under the heading "Interventions to challenge and modify fusion meta-beliefs".

Note

1 The title MCTI® Registered Therapist ascertains that the therapist has successfully completed adequate training in MCT, i.e. the MCTI® Masterclass training. A list of MCTI® registered therapists in different countries can be found at www.mct-institute.co.uk.

4   The treatment, Part II

Modifying the metacognitive beliefs

Interventions to modify metacognitive beliefs about uncontrollability

Meta-beliefs about repetitive negative thinking as something uncontrollable are challenged in the explorative dialogue between therapist and client and with the help of interventions such as *detached mindfulness* (DM) and postponement of worry and rumination. Exercises and meta-cognitive behavioral experiments are preceded by verbal interventions. Verbal reattribution, and the exploration and challenging about worry as uncontrollable could look like this:

T: *Do you worry all the time intensively or are there also moments when you don't?*

P: It can be quite calm sometimes. It is only when things happen or could happen that the worry increases. The worry often comes when I have this lump in my stomach, and when I feel that something could have happened to my children.

T: *In those instances, do you feel that the worry takes you by surprise?*

P: Pretty much so, yes.

T: *Like you can't choose whether to worry or not?*

P: No, in those situations the worry is impossible to control.

T: *But if something were to happen around you at the same time. If your sister called you and said she had an accident and needed your immediate assistance to get to the hospital. What would you do then?*

P: Then of course I put everything aside and would have full focus on helping her as soon as possible.

T: *You would not ask her to wait because you were busy worrying?*

P: Ugh, no, of course not. In such a situation, I would obviously throw myself away and come to her assistance.

T: *So, in such a situation, you could decide to help your sister instead of continuing the worry process? What does that say about worry as either uncontrollable or perfectly controllable?*

P: Well, then it's the tense situation that makes me distracted, not me who chooses or controls.

DOI: 10.4324/9781003597100-5

T: *What do you make of this? That it is the situations that distract you or that it is you who then make different priorities and that it would be you who would choose to prioritize, for example, your sister over your thoughts in a situation where she needs your immediate assistance?*

P: Of course, you can see it as me prioritizing her needs over my own thoughts.

T: *So, worry can be about what you prioritize when paying attention, rather than something that just comes over you in certain situations? Do you still believe that your worry is 95 percent uncontrollable?*

Verbal interventions to challenge the meta-belief of uncontrollability are followed up by behavioral experiments and exercises. Detached mindfulness (DM) and postponement of worry are alternative strategies that clients with worry problems are introduced to. Clients with depressive problems and a high degree of rumination are introduced both to DM, postponement of rumination and attention exercises such as the *attention training technique* (ATT) or the *spatial attention control exercise* (SpACE). DM is described in more detail in the second next paragraph, ATT and SpACE later in this chapter. All these interventions are designed to reduce worry and rumination and to radically reduce uncontrollability beliefs.

Thought suppression experiments

"For the next minute, you can think of whatever you want, except a blue polar bear". In MCT, this is often introduced as an initial experiment in the case of worry problems after the case formulation and socialization to the model has been done. The experiment is usually carried out before detached mindfulness (DM) is introduced. What usually happens is that the client discovers that thought suppression is a counterproductive strategy that strengthens the belief that worry is uncontrollable and that it is also a rather energy-consuming strategy. The client usually recognizes himself or herself having used thought suppression to try to deal with negative thoughts and that this has contributed to the negative thought processes being perceived as both uncontrollable and dangerous. The experiment is also used to highlight that detached mindfulness (DM) is something qualitatively different.

Detached mindfulness (DM)

If the problems according to MCT are caused, intensified and maintained by the CAS, the obvious solution is to cancel CAS and to stop the repetitive negative thinking. CAS means a response to the trigger, an engagement in the trigger. Is it possible to refrain from engaging in negative thoughts instead? Can you not respond to trigger thoughts? If you still believe that the trigger thoughts can bring some important messages, can you still postpone engaging in them until a short while later in the day? The antithesis of CAS is detached mindfulness (DM). DM means noting a thought as separate from the observing self and for the moment doing nothing with it (Wells, 2005b, 2009).

DM is not the same as Buddhist-inspired mindfulness. DM is a more accurate concept and refers only to the relationship and approach to a thought. Unlike much of what is usually meant by Buddhist-inspired mindfulness, when practicing DM, you don't have to bother about how you breathe, whether you're here and now or not, or whether you look at the events around you as if they occurred for the first time in your life. Rather, all such instructions are discouraged. DM is not about developing new rituals for dealing with thoughts. To practice DM, you do not need to meditate for 45 minutes every day for several weeks. DM is an immediate and straightforward act, or rather a non-act. To try to look at events as if you yourself were a tabula rasa, new to all impressions, would in MCT be seen as overcomplicating and as an indication that an engagement in thoughts is ongoing. Similar instructions could also lead to an increased degree of self-focused attention.

DM is thus noting a thought and doing nothing with it. Techniques that can be used in other psychotherapy approaches, such as imagining placing a negative thought on a leaf and then letting it float away with the current, are something different from DM. Based on MCT, the objection would be: "Is that doing nothing with a thought or doing something with it?"

Introducing and further applying DM

There are several ways to introduce and start practicing DM as an alternative strategy to CAS. It's like noticing the thought, taking a step back in the mind, and then letting the thought take care of itself. It is to see the thought from the outside, to separate oneself from it instead of being in the thought and instead of looking at your life from the inside of the thought. An example of seeing your life from the inside of a thought could be "I am a complete failure" and at the same time relate to oneself and to the world around you as if this were a fact, an actual problem and not a thought. One way to introduce detached mindfulness (DM) could look like this:

T: *Your idea that you are a complete failure, do you think it's possible to stop engaging in it? In MCT, we have a term for this: "detached mindfulness", abbreviated to "DM", which means to only note a thought, but for the moment doing nothing with it.*

P: It would be a relief, but it is there in the back of my mind, and it follows me wherever I go, pretty much all the time. I just can't get rid of it.

T: *Are you trying to get rid of that thought?*

P: Yes, but as I just said, I just can't get rid of it. It keeps on coming back to me.

T: *Do you think it is possible to try to get rid of the thought without you getting involved in it at the same time?*

P: No, of course, I get very preoccupied with wanting and trying to get rid of it ...

T: *Have you tried not to do anything at all with the thought? To detach yourself from it? Can you try right now for a while just to note the thought that you are a failure without either trying to remove it or to respond to it?*

The different ways to introduce DM are:

1 To make the client aware of times when she on a daily basis and naturally applies DM to most thoughts, even if the client has so far probably not called this approach "detached mindfulness".
2 Through metaphors.
3 Through experience-based exercises and metacognitive behavioral experiments.

When the client is made aware that DM is a skill that most of us already possess and practice naturally every day, the dialogue can begin with a discussion about the number of thoughts that pass through our mind every day, something like this:

T: *How many thoughts did you have yesterday, do you think?*
P: That is hard to say, but I guess it was thousands.
T: *Do you remember all the thoughts from yesterday?*
P: No, it's probably only a few, if any.
T: *Where are all those thoughts now?*
P: ?
T: *Could you conclude that you have let go of most of the thoughts from yesterday, just left them behind? That you somehow have applied detached mindfulness?*

Most of the thoughts from yesterday are of course no longer present in our conscious mind. Somehow, we have left them behind. Hardly ever, probably never, do we consider how we go about when we leave them behind, for example, the thought of how we tied our shoelaces yesterday morning. We just leave the thought. It's hard to explain how that process works, exactly how to go about leaving a thought behind. The best answer is probably "I didn't do anything with the thought and what happened then was that it somehow left my consciousness by itself". If you were to be asked why you didn't continue to process the idea of how to tie your shoes, the question would most likely be perceived as absurd, but the answer would probably be that this thought is so unimportant that it could safely be left to its own fate. Somehow, a metacognitive process seems to be going on where thoughts are appraised as more or less important and where DM is applied naturally to the thoughts that are perceived as fully managed and then meaningless to go on with.

Anyone who has experienced worry and rumination as uncontrollable processes may discover that control over the CAS could be reformulated into a question of priorities and choices being made among different thoughts, as important or unimportant to engage in.

The dialogue about natural occasions of DM can then turn into a dialogue about whether it may be possible to apply DM in relation to all thoughts. Possibly, it may first be necessary to verbally challenge the difference between significant and insignificant thoughts. Someone may object that a certain failure in life has had a huge impact and is associated with a completely different emotional charge and therefore cannot in any way be equated with thoughts about how shoelaces are tied. Follow-up questions in a metacognitive exploration could then be: "Even if the failure was very painful for you then, does that mean that thoughts about it are important today? Who is it that makes the evaluation and categorization of certain thoughts more important than others? In what way does a thought become more significant if it coexists with a certain emotion? Could it be that you are always still in control of your thought processes and that you choose to engage in the thoughts you find important to deal with and choose to let go of others?" At the same time, note that questions such as those in the example above are not asked at the same time or directly after each other. Instead, the dialogue should be characterized by explorative questions that are asked one at a time and which the client is then given the opportunity to reflect on and give feedback on.

Various metaphors are also used to introduce DM. "You usually can't choose if someone should knock on your front door, but who is it that decides whether you should open it or not? It is not possible to decide whether your phone should ring, but can you choose not to answer? When the trigger thought knocks or rings, can you choose not to answer it?" "If you still think it might have something important to tell you, can you ask it to call back a little later?" Another metaphor could be that of sitting in a forest clearing in the spring and watching birds. "Are you trying to control what the birds are going to do, which of them is going to land and where, who is going to fly on and when? Or do you just look at them as a passive spectator and see what they come up with? Maybe you lose interest in them after a while and let your gaze wander towards something else. Can you do the same with your thoughts?" Again, and as pointed out in the previous paragraph, metaphors as well as the explorative questions associated with them should be given one at a time with room for reflection, not several in succession.

Metaphors about DM are followed up by exercises and experiments. For example, the therapist might suggest an experiential exercise like this:

T: *Can we both try to just sit quietly for a minute or so and observe what thoughts pop into our minds? Try not to control or edit the thoughts. Instead, take a step back into your mind and take note of what comes up.*

P: [When the minute has passed] I found it difficult. I don't know if I really understood what I was supposed to do. I didn't really manage to catch my thoughts.

T: *What did you do when you got the idea that you didn't really understand? Did you start to get involved in that thought in some way?*

P: I was probably most stressed and felt a bit stupid.

T: *How did you go about trying to capture your thoughts? Were you detached at the time or were you getting involved in your thoughts?*

P: No, I was probably not detached from my thoughts, I think, rather engaged in them.

T: *Can we do the test one more time? If you should have a thought that you have not understood the exercise, can you try to just note that thought among all the other thoughts?*

The client needs to be given the opportunity to discover the difference between simply noticing a thought and engaging with it. Talking your way to it or trying to grasp it by intensive and prolonged thinking, will have obvious limitations, in the same way that there are limitations to trying to think about what, for example, dancing, an itchy mosquito bite or humor is. It is probably not DM, but just more thinking you engage with when you try to analyze if you really understand the concept. MCT sessions therefore contain many exercises and metacognitive experiments where the therapist guides and where the client and therapist then examine the client's experiences of DM. "Was it possible to do nothing with the negative thought or did you still do something to control it?" The exercises are often repeated after short feedback from the client. The purpose of repeated exercises is for the client to gain an increasingly correct understanding and clearer experiences of DM. Another purpose of the exercises may be to give the client the opportunity to identify more and more trigger thoughts. For example, during the exercises, you may discover that you also have trigger thoughts about your emotions, such as "Now my anxiety is approaching an intolerable level".

Summaries and feedback after the exercises aim at increased generalization and broader application of DM. What happens during the MCT session can be seen as model situations for how the client should be able to practice DM outside the sessions and in their daily life. When the client describes an experience of detached mindfulness during the session, this is often followed up by questions such as: "Is this how you usually deal with your negative thoughts? Are there any thoughts that you can't apply DM to? How can you practice this in the coming week?"

Another DM exercise is to role-play with negative thoughts. A client with OCD, for example, may take on the role of obsessive thoughts while the therapist assumes the role of DM. The role-play and experiment could be carried out like this:

T: *Your obsessions often tell you that you still have remnants of feces on your hands, even though you really know you're clean enough, right?*

P: Yes, it's hard and I just get more and more stressed when I start washing myself and changing clothes.

T: *My suggestion is that we try a DM exercise.*

P: Well, okay, I guess.

T: *If we try a role-play for a while and I'm you noticing your obsessive thoughts.*

P: ?

T: *And if you would like to let your usual obsessions speak to me and command me. Are you keeping up?*

P: You mean that I should say all the things to you that the obsessive thoughts usually tell me?

T: *That's right. And then I'll see if I can apply DM when I hear the obsessive thoughts. Can we get started?*

P: Yes, okay then. But it feels horrible and very embarrassing to say these things to you, but okay. You already know roughly how they can sound.

T: *Yes, that's right.*

P: Okay, I'll get started: You can feel your hands, they're not clean yet!

T: *Well, I can hear you say that.*

P: Yes, but do you really listen? You still have poop residue left on your hands. It's really disgusting.

T: Oh, yes? Anything else you want to tell me?

P: Yes, I told you that you must wash your hands once again. More properly this time!

T: Oh, yes?

P: But don't you listen? You're not clean!

T: I remember you said something about it just a moment ago, yes.

P: Yes, and it's important because you still have poop residue on your hands, which you risk smudging around when you get dressed and go into the kitchen.

T: Mmm.

P: You don't seem to listen or take this seriously!

After the exercise, the therapist asks how it felt to be in the role of obsessive thought. "Pretty hard, right? Like speaking to someone who isn't listening?" One conclusion is often that it is much more demanding to be a nagging obsession than to be the one who applies DM. The exercise is then repeated, but with reversed roles and preferably with additional trigger thoughts, such as "You only dare to ignore the dirty thoughts when you are together with the therapist. You will never dare to do this at home!". Other questions from the therapist in connection with various DM exercises aimed at generalizing effects and modifying uncontrollability beliefs can be: "What is it you have actually tried? Can you describe it as a new way of relating to your thoughts? You will have your thoughts as your company wherever you go, won't you? If you could refrain from responding to your thoughts here with me during the exercise, don't you always have that ability? Could it be that your worry has always been and always will be completely controllable? Maybe the problem was that you *believed* you couldn't control it?"

Further and more detailed descriptions of the concept of DM and more experience-based DM exercises are described in Wells (2005b, 2009).

Postponement of worry and rumination

Combined with DM, the client is also introduced to postponement of worry and/or rumination. Instead of engaging in trigger thoughts for long periods of the day, this is about limiting repetitive negative thinking, getting used to interrupting the negative thought process, and instead setting aside short moments when you can engage with the thoughts. It is emphasized to the client that the worry time/thinking time is then voluntary and that the point of the experiment is precisely to explore whether the engagement in the thoughts can be postponed. The instruction is usually that the worry or rumination time should be 10 minutes long, not in connection with bedtime in the evening, but sometime at the end of the day and preferably at a fixed time. If the client should object that 10 minutes sounds too little, this will be discussed. The objection may be formulated as a new trigger and new concern: "Of course, one can also worry about such a thing. Can you try to postpone your response to that thought until the worry time as well? If 10 minutes were to be perceived as too short, is it possible to postpone the rest of the worry to tomorrow's thinking time?"

Worry-postponing is to be seen as a metacognitive behavioral experiment. At the next therapy session, the homework assignment is followed up. You discuss how it has all worked out, whether it has been possible at all or only at certain moments or with certain thoughts. The therapist explores in detail when and with which triggers the postponement has worked, and in addition, if there have been other trigger thoughts, perhaps associated with special negative emotions where the client has found it more difficult to postpone worry. If, which is unusual, the client should say that the postponement has not worked at all, the reasons for this are of course explored. Has the client even tried? Possible reasons are that the client has confused trigger with worry, anxiety with worry or stress with worry. A client who has found worry postponement difficult could say: "I have tried to postpone, but it has not worked, the thoughts have been present anyway". Something that needs to be clarified in that case is that what was intended was postponement of *the response* to the thoughts and the therapist could then ask: "But even if the thoughts were there, could you postpone your response to them?"

Further exploration of situations where the client describes that worry or rumination postponement has not worked, usually indicates that the client has used other strategies than DM, such as thought suppression. For example, the therapist might ask, "When you noticed that the thoughts continued to be there, what did you do? Was it just as a passive observation or were you trying to get rid of them somehow?" An explorative dialogue about how the homework task of applying DM and postponement has worked, could look like this:

T: *You say that it has only partly worked to practice DM and to postpone worry. Can you tell me about the last time you tried and felt that it didn't work?*

P: Last night it was difficult. I started worrying again about whether my girlfriend might be planning to break up with me. I didn't dare to ask her again, because I know how nagging she thinks I can be and then I just get even more worried that she will break up.

T: *So, what was the trigger thought? "Is she going to break up?"*

P: Something like that, or maybe rather "What if she's getting tired of me".

T: *Did you try to postpone your worry?*

P: Yes, and for a short while I probably succeeded.

T: *And what happened next?*

P: Hmm, it's a bit funny, but after a while I probably started to investigate whether the thought had really disappeared.

T: *And what happened then?*

P: Well, then it came back of course.

T: *That searching for the trigger doesn't really sound like leaving the thought alone, do you agree? My suggestion now is that we try one more exercise to see how you could apply DM and worry postponement also in a situation like this.*

Before any agreement is reached at all on the postponement experiment, the purpose needs to be clear. If the case formulation has previously made it evident that worry or rumination causes significant problems in the client's life, the purpose of the experiment usually appears crystal clear, i.e. that it is about exploring whether it is possible to significantly reduce worry and rumination through postponement. The worry/rumination time is therefore voluntary. If the client forgets about it or would rather do something else during that moment of the day, then this is completely in line with the experiment. Sometimes the therapist is asked if it's recommended that the client take notes of their trigger thoughts in case they should have been forgotten when the worry time occurs. A counter-question can then be: "If you risk forgetting the thought, how important do you think it is?" Another counter-question could be: "If you worry about forgetting a thought, can you try to also postpone that worry until your worry time as well?" The important thing is to consistently try to postpone the involvement in trigger thoughts. If the client thinks they may be important, there is still the opportunity to find out whether the thoughts are still perceived as important after some hours of postponement. Most adults can relate to postponement or making appointments for important or even unimportant meetings. If you want, you can look at the postponement like arranging a meeting with yourself at the end of the day and before that noting to yourself "there was a trigger, I'll deal with it at 19.00 if necessary". Of course, it is also possible to use the analogy of watching a movie: "I'll pause the movie right now and can continue watching it at 7:00 p.m. if I want to".

When the CAS is activated during the therapy session, on co-rumination and "co-worrying" between client and therapist

When the client's long-term problems can be conceptualized in terms of repetitive negative thinking along with other CAS activity, it would of course be unexpected if these processes did not also appear in the interaction between client and therapist. As well as rumination can carry on privately in our own mind, two people, something that was also mentioned in the previous chapter, can have conversations that clearly could be characterized as rumination, or rather as co-rumination (see, for example, Spendelow et al., 2017). A client with worry problems can of course worry about whether MCT is the right form of therapy, whether their own problem is treatable or whether they have understood the meaning of, for example, DM in the correct way. Someone might worry about things like "who will I be if I stop worrying completely" or "what am I going to do with all the time that I used to spend worrying?" Asking for reassurance is a common behavior when dealing with worry. Sometimes reassurance questions are directed to the therapist: "What do you think? Do you think I'll be able to manage this new job? Do you think I will make progress in this therapy?" A treatment in which the client and therapist spend long periods of time worrying or ruminating together, or where the therapist consistently gives reassurance, is devastating for the outcome of the treatment and adds nothing qualitatively new for the patient. For the treatment to be effective, the client needs to be helped to recognize when the CAS is activated and to interrupt and postpone worry and rumination. Tendencies to ask for reassurance need to be conceptualized and labeled as elements of the CAS. Something that has already been emphasized: The therapist needs to be so familiar with the model that they detect when CAS is activated during the session and during an ongoing conversation. The therapist needs to respond on a different level and be able to switch the dialogue from the object level to the metacognitive level. Many of the interventions in MCT are therefore used directly when CAS is activated in the dialogue during the session. An example of a patient with rumination problems could look like this:

P: Okay, now I've tried to postpone my analysis until later, but I don't understand how that can be of any help for me. I have tried most of the current existing medications and different therapies and I feel that this will not be able to help either. It all feels hopeless. Also, it is quite superficial. I've had these problems for so many years and I think that they have left such traces in my brain that everything is already too late. Or at least something completely different would be needed. Maybe psychoanalysis or hypnosis or even some sort of system reboot like ECT, Psilocybin, or something. This technique of postponing thoughts will simply not be able to solve my problems.

T: *It seems like a lot of thinking is going on right now and as a result your feelings of hopeless deepens and you come to conclusions that it's all too late? Doesn't it look like rumination what you're doing right now? Can we see if it's possible to do nothing with these thoughts for a little while? Maybe we can come back to the question of whether this will help or not and for now instead follow the agenda for the session and try another exercise in detached mindfulness?*

Can worry and rumination ever become uncontrollable?

Another behavioral experiment to challenge uncontrollability meta-beliefs, is the "loss of control experiment". This experiment is not carried out until a bit later in the treatment when the client has had experiences of DM and postponement of worry. In the experiment, the client is asked to increase the worry during the session, and later as a homework assignment, to such intense levels that it becomes uncontrollable. Before the experiment is carried out, the therapist and client discuss what proofs to look for that could lead to the conclusion that worry has indeed become uncontrollable. After the test, when the client has been encouraged to push worry until it gets uncontrollable, the result is considered. Was it possible to lose control of the worry? If not, how come? If the client's anxiety would have increased in connection with the intense worry, or perhaps rather the worry that the experiment would lead to something bad, does that mean that the worry has gone uncontrollable? Is it ever possible to lose control of your worry?

Among clients with worry or rumination problems, it is not uncommon to have uncontrollability beliefs such as "once I've started to worry, it is impossible to interrupt" or "once I am stuck in rumination, I cannot get out of it". Similar exercises to the uncontrollability experiment can then be carried out where the client is encouraged to worry or ruminate intensely for one or a few minutes and then interrupt the thought process and apply DM. After that, the worry or rumination can be pushed again and after a while interrupted again. Summarizing and evaluative dialogues about the experiment revolve around whether the worry or rumination became uncontrollable and why it did not. A prerequisite for these experiments is that the client has already gained sufficient experience and a correct understanding of

DM. The therapist's hypothesis is that worry, and rumination can never become uncontrollable, and that the client always has the option to interrupt worry and rumination.

The purpose of a behavioral experiment such as pushing worry until it becomes uncontrollable is thus to challenge the meta-belief of uncontrollability. Even if the client reports anxiety during or after the experiment, if necessary, the therapist will remind the client of the previous case formulation, and the distinction already made between worry and anxiety. A person with worry and anxiety problems may worry about their anxiety, about whether the anxiety will get too intense and whether it can become unbearable or become almost constant and debilitating. In that case, it needs to be made clear that worry about increasing anxiety becomes an additional worry theme and that the trigger thoughts about anxiety are ones that the client can choose to either engage in or apply DM to. The point is to expose the meta-belief that the worry may become uncontrollable to a test. Before negative meta-beliefs about danger are to be challenged and modified, uncontrollability beliefs about worry and rumination need to approach zero. The therapist follows this up using the weekly scales and through continuous ratings of meta-beliefs before and after the interventions used.

Exercises to facilitate increased flexibility and executive control of attention

In for example depressive states, attention can appear "locked" in rumination, pessimism, hopelessness and threat monitoring of symptoms, emotions and motivation. Several attention techniques have been developed (see for example Wells, 2009) to redirect attention away from rumination, worry and threat monitoring. The exercises aim to modify metacognitive beliefs and to increase executive control over attention. They are also used to facilitate more flexible use of attention. As with other interventions, the various attention exercises are introduced after the case formulation and socialization is completed. That is, the exercises should follow logically from a case formulation where therapist and client have jointly identified how persistent and persevering threat-focused attention leads to symptom development and worsening of symptoms.

The techniques are not about distraction from negative thoughts or about avoiding negative emotions. Regarding distraction, which is conceptualized as a CAS strategy, the goal there seems to be thought suppression, i.e. a strategy to shift attentional focus to shut out and get rid of negative thoughts and feelings. A problematic effect of thought suppression and distraction is that you continue to relate to negative thoughts, continue to make them important and thus be reminded of them more frequently. To try to push away thoughts is to relate to them and to be in continued contact with them. Distraction is an ineffective coping strategy, which those who experience emotional problems are usually painfully aware of.

The attentional exercises in MCT are qualitatively and functionally different from distraction, emotion control and thought suppression. Refocusing during various attention exercises in MCT does not constitute responses to trigger thoughts, does not aim to relate to them or to erase them from consciousness. The negative thoughts are allowed to remain as long as they do, the client is encouraged to only note them if they appear in the consciousness, but for the moment focus on something else. Nor do the exercises aim to manage or control negative emotions. Instead, refocusing is about the fact that at every moment of our lives, we receive visual stimuli, sounds, tastes and smells from our surroundings and a continuous stream of impressions from our bodies, so-called interoceptive stimuli. Concepts such as selective perception and attention control describe how we make choices between the impressions and thoughts we direct our focus towards and those we stop and dwell on. Unlike distraction, refocusing is rather about "Sure, there's a negative thought again, but right now I'm letting it be and focusing on x instead" or "Yes I know, I don't feel happy right now, but now I'm focusing on y instead for a moment". That is, a negative thought is only *one* possible stimulus to let one's attention dwell on, but there are also many, many other choices at any given moment.

The attention exercises are used to interrupt and reduce rumination, worry, and threat monitoring. By radically reducing the time spent on worry and rumination, cognitive resources are released for other changes to take place. It will be easier for the client to focus on work, studies and social relationships, including participating actively in a constructive and explorative dialogue during the therapy session. It becomes easier to realize that life can be lived even with negative thoughts and feelings. The thoughts do not need to be dealt with, waited out or made to disappear. The focus can be directed towards other events, preferably towards events that are more fun, important and interesting. The attention exercises also aim to change metacognitive beliefs about uncontrollability. A person who is depressed and initially ruminates a lot may perceive rumination as biologically controlled, controlled by depression itself rather than by metacognitive beliefs.

Attention training technique (ATT)

Attention training technique (ATT) (see for example Wells, 2009) is an exercise, about 12 minutes long, where you actively listen to different sounds that are presented at the same time and that come from several directions. During the exercise, the client is guided to shift attention between the different sounds and between the different spatial locations from which the sounds originate. Should negative thoughts arise about their own performance in relation to the exercise or negative thoughts about the exercise itself, the client is encouraged to relate to these as to additional sounds in the soundscape. The client's experience of internal attention versus external attention is rated before and after the exercise, with an expectation that the focus of attention will be more external. The rating is based on a scale between minus 3 (entirely externally focused) and plus 3 (entirely self-focused). The client is expected to have moved at least two steps towards the external direction after the exercise. If this has not happened, the therapist explores in the subsequent dialogue what may have prevented this. The client is then prescribed to carry out these exercises daily for a period. The purpose of the exercise is to interrupt persevering thought processes and to increase the experience of executive control over attention. Another goal of the exercise is for the client to be able to use their attention more flexibly to external events in the environment instead of predominantly towards negative feelings and thoughts. The purpose is neither relaxation, nor the avoidance of negative emotions. The exercise is intended to be carried out regardless of the current mood, emotions and symptoms. ATT is usually included as one intervention among several in MCT. There is an original recording of ATT that is copyrighted for research purposes and that is no longer available for clinicians in MCT training or supervision. Instead, many registered MCT therapists, as well as therapists in MCT training, are doing ATT with their natural ongoing sounds, but with the same setup and instructions as described. An introduction of ATT and a follow-up dialogue after the exercise could go like this:

P: But I just can't free myself from thinking about everything I've destroyed and how worthless I am. The thoughts haunt me and torment me all the time! What should I do really? I am confused. I don't even know if it's worth continuing this treatment.

T: *Should we try an exercise that is designed to make it easier to free oneself from negative thought patterns?*

P: But I really don't know if it's the right thing for me. I suspect that it will feel like just another hopeless thing to try.

T: *My suggestion is that we try and then we can talk further afterwards about how it turned out and if it can be helpful.*

P: Mmm, okay.

T: *I will ask you to direct your attention to different sounds that are going on at the same time here and now. What sounds can you hear around you right now?*

P: Well, I can hear the computer over there buzzing, the clock on the wall to my left ticking, and then I can hear something mumbling from the room next to yours. Then of course I hear some cars passing by outside the window and every now and then some kind of tractor or excavator or whatever it is.

T: *Then we have some sounds that we make use of. Before we get started, may I ask you where your focus of attention is right now? If you were to estimate between minus 3 and plus 3, where minus 3 is totally external, towards events around you and plus 3 indicates that your attention is totally internal, self-focused towards your thoughts and feelings?*

P: Maybe plus 2 then.

T: *[After guiding the client around with varied attention focus between the different sounds and spatial locations for 12 minutes according to the ATT instruction] Did you hear all the sounds when I asked you to listen to them?*

P: Most of the time. But once when you asked me to listen to the excavator out there, it just happened to be quiet.

T: *How would you rate your attention on the scale right now?*

P: Maybe plus 0.5 then.

T: *[Had expected the client to move at least two steps towards the external direction and suspects that the client may have started to worry or ruminate during the exercise] Okay, the excavator was quiet when you were asked to listen to it, but was it still possible to listen for that sound?*

P: Yes.

T: *Did you ever lose concentration?*

P: Yes, several times. I'm probably not good at this. Maybe I'm in too bad shape right now. I don't think my brain can handle it really.

T: *Tell me, what happened when you lost focus?*

P: I noticed that I started to think about whether I felt too bad to be able to do exercises like this after all, and suddenly I was far away from the exercise.

T: *Ah, so you started to ruminate and think about whether you feel too bad to manage this?*

P: Yes, that's pretty much how my thoughts went.

T: *I would like to suggest to you to do this exercise twice daily at home. If you have negative thoughts during the exercise, such as the thoughts that you are in too bad shape to manage the task, would it be possible to relate to the thoughts as to just another sound in the soundscape? Just note them like noise and move your attention on to the next sound?*

Before the exercise, the therapist may ask the client to record the exercise and then to listen to the recording daily at home. Alternatively, therapist and client can together plan for a similar situation at home where, daily, the client shifts their attention between different sounds from different spatial locations. The therapist asks questions about the client's experience of control over attention during the exercise, such as: "This moving your attention around in this way, is that something that you always have control over? No matter what happens to you in life and what happens to you internally?" That is, the key here is that the client is given the opportunity to discover that the focus of attention is independent of both external and internal events. The client thus gains experience of being able to focus on what they want regardless of external and internal stimuli. This experience is at the heart of self-regulation.

There are also studies that have shown positive effects of ATT as a stand-alone treatment for various anxiety and depression disorders (Knowles et al., 2016), reduced self-focus in worry and anxiety (Fergus & Wheless,

2018), reduced frequency of intrusive thoughts after stressful life events (Nassif & Wells, 2014), reduced stress and meta-worry in college students (Myhr et al., 2019), neurophysiological changes associated with increased attention control (Knowles & Wells, 2018), and that ATT on one occasion seems to have led to increased ability of 5–6-year-old children to postpone a reward until later (Murray et al., 2016, 2018).

Spatial attention control exercise (SpACE)

SpACE is an alternative exercise to ATT but has the same purpose. During the exercise, the client is instructed to alternately focus on sounds from different directions, on sounds that may be present in the area to the left of the client, to the right, behind and in front. The exercise aims to increase awareness of thoughts as well as flexible control over attention, and to ensure that this control is experienced as independent of both internal events such as thoughts and feelings, and external events. The therapist uses the practice to strengthen adaptive metacognition and to modify meta-beliefs about uncontrollability. The technique is briefly described in, for example, Wells et al. (2021).

Situational attentional refocusing (SAR)

In cases of problems with, for example, social anxiety or post-traumatic stress, this technique is used. SAR has partly different purposes than ATT. If ATT aims to interrupt persevering thought processes, SAR is designed to extend information processing to other events that are available in the situation and that are not perceived as threat related. In the case of social anxiety, SAR exercises are designed where the client experiments with shifting focus away from monitoring "self as social object" and externally towards the environment, towards how other people in a social situation are dressed or what eye color they have, how the timbre of their voices sound or what they are talking about. In the case of post-traumatic stress, exercises may involve interrupting threat monitoring for a while and instead paying attention to signals in the environment that convey information that the situation currently appears to be normal and sufficiently safe. As well as scanning for critical faces or potentially judging people in your environment, you can try to look for those who look neutral or even interested and friendly. (More about the concept of "self as social object" in social anxiety and about CAS and metacognitive beliefs in PTSD are described in chapters 5 and 6.) An exercise with a client with PTSD symptoms could go something like this:

T: *Isn't it always possible to find potential dangers if you search for them? Here in these premises, for example, how many things do you see around you that could possibly endanger our life?*

P: Well, the electrical plugs may not be brand new. It could start a fire.

T: *And more?*

P: I don't know what kind of people there are in the rest of the clinic here. One of them out in the waiting room could be a terrorist who is currently planning to rush in here with a large knife in his hand.

T: *Theoretically, that's not completely impossible of course.*

P: Some violent crazy drug addict, like the one who knocked me down, could kick in the front door out there, rush in here and start beating us.

T: *Mmm.*

P: An airliner could crash into the house here tanked up with fuel.

T: *Yes, if you start looking for dangers, you will easily find them, isn't that true?*

P: Yes, and that's probably what I do almost all the time.

T: *But if this is a choice you make, to look for possible dangers, is it possible to turn your attention to something else instead?*

P: Yes, but I feel so scared and insecure all the time.

T: *But do you think that your attention depends on how you feel?*

P: Well, that is of course my experience ...

T: *Would it instead be possible to watch for everything in here that signals that the situation seems normal and even safe?*

P: Well, the windows are not broken and it's warm and nice here.

T: *Anything else?*

P: Yes, you are friendly and seem to be caring and nice. The people out there in the waiting room looked like ordinary people.

T: *Did you now have a feeling that you could choose your focus for attention?*

P: Yes, I could.

T: *Do you think that what you do with your attention has consequences for your emotional well-being?*

Note that an exercise such as the one in the example above does not aim at distraction from anxiety. Instead, the therapist tried to help the client discover that they can flexibly choose their focus of attention and that it becomes very difficult to move forward in life and to feel safe if you are constantly checking for dangers.

Similarly, refocusing attention can be used with someone who is persistently focused on the loss of a relationship. The therapist could then ask: "Just as you can think about what you have lost and that you feel so lonely and abandoned, can you also focus for a moment on new opportunities that could appear? For example, do you have more opportunities now to develop your own interests? New chances to find new relationships? Can you turn your attention now for a while to the new possible opportunities?" A client who worries about giving a presentation or a talk can be encouraged to shift focus: "If you detach for a moment from the thought that a few people in the audience might be critical of your presentation, can you instead direct your attention to what you would like to convey? To what you think is most interesting and most important in what you are going to present? Can you for a moment convey to me what you find most interesting?" A person who is dreading important decisions and worries that others might be disappointed or upset might be asked: "Just as you may worry about disappointing and upsetting others when you make your decision, is it possible for a moment, instead to direct your attention to what you would like to achieve by the decision and in what way it is important to you?" The client can be instructed to shift attentional focus a few times between thoughts of the loss or what might be scary and to the possibilities. Again, in these examples, the purpose would not be distraction from negative thoughts and feelings, but instead increased executive control of attention and more flexible use of it.

To further illustrate the possibilities with attentional refocusing, what follows is a fictitious dialogue and exercise with a client with study- and concentration problems:

T: *What do you think, how come you find it so difficult to effectively prepare before an exam?*

P: I'm not sure, but I think it might be some kind of attention deficit disorder that I suffer from. I'm easily distracted by other things when I'm studying, and I take way too many and too long breaks.

T: *What could it be that is distracting you? Can you guide me through the last time this happened?*

P: Well, a new course started this Monday but when I opened the book at home, I got completely exhausted and restless when I realized how many pages there were and how compact the text was.

T: *What might have been the trigger thought? Is this going to be too difficult? What if I don't pass the course?*

P: I think both of those thoughts might have been present. I probably started to worry that I wouldn't pass the course and that I wouldn't be able to stick to my study discipline. I was also distracted by feeling so dull and restless.

T: *Was the problem that you were unconcentrated, do you think, or could it have been that you on the contrary were very concentrated, but on the wrong events?*

P: When you put it that way ... Of course, I became very involved in the thoughts of failure.

T: *Can we try an attention exercise where I ask you to read a passage from that thick book on psychology that I have on my bookshelf? Do you think the text is somewhat complicated to get through?*

P: Yes, it doesn't look too easy to get through.

T: *I would like to ask for your permission to be your negative thoughts while you read. The task for you will then be to alternate between listening to what I say and focusing as best you can on reading and trying to understand what you read. All right?*

P: What do you mean by being my thoughts?

T: *If I may speak your negative thoughts out loud when you are reading? Like trying to distract you when you are reading.*

P: Okay, we can try. Should I start reading here?

T: *[After the client has started reading aloud] Keep reading and focus on what I'm saying at the same time. What I have to say is very important now. "I don't think you understand what you're reading right now. It's going too slowly. You also seem very unfocused now. You seem to show obvious ADHD problems". And now for a moment, shift your focus as much as possible to what you are reading and to understanding the text as best you can. Don't let yourself be distracted by what I'm saying. [T continues to verbalize the negative thoughts.]*

Interventions to modify danger metacognitive beliefs

As meta-beliefs about uncontrollability drop and approach zero, something often happens with the danger metacognitive beliefs as well. These also tend to decrease. This can probably be understood in the sense that if you have previously worried that worry may harm your physical or mental health and no longer believe that worry is uncontrollable, there will be no point to worrying about the hypothetical dangers of worry. The experience now is that there are effective ways to interrupt worry and rumination.

Historical evidence of the danger of worry/rumination

As with the modification of uncontrollability beliefs, the work begins by verbally challenging the danger meta-beliefs. This can be done through dialogues about historical data that could provide support for the belief, for example such as this:

T: *How many times have you worried that your worry will make you lose your mind?*

P: Oh, I must have worried about that a hundred or even thousands of times.

T: *Has it happened so far?*

P: I've had problems with anxiety and worry for most of my life … but no, yet I haven't gone crazy at any time as far as I know.

T: *You've worried for most of your life and even about losing your mind, probably hundreds or even thousands of times, but so far you haven't lost your mind. What do you make of that? How much do you now believe that continued worry can drive you crazy?*

Mechanism explanations regarding the danger of worry/rumination

The verbal challenge of danger meta-beliefs is also done by asking for mechanism explanations. Such a dialogue could go like this:

T: *You've told me that you believe that your worries can cause burnout and even damage your brain. If so, what do you think happens when worry damages a brain? How exactly would that come about?*

P: I don't really know. I'm not a doctor or psychologist, but I've read that stress can damage the brain. My stress increases when I'm worried and I think I've read and heard that high stress levels over a long period of time can damage the brain. For example, I have heard about various stress hormones that are released and that can damage the body and brain if they do not return to normal levels.

T: *In what way would that happen, do you think? If you consider evolution and human existence in previous eras. How do you think Stone Age people felt about stress? Or people who survived the Black Death? Shouldn't their stress levels have been high? Should we guess that they were brain damaged by stress or that stress is rather a reaction that in dire situations has promoted survival in humans and other mammals?*

Behavioral experiments to challenge and modify danger metacognitive beliefs

Verbal interventions are followed by metacognitive behavioral experiments. One such scenario could be, for example, asking a person with generalized anxiety disorder to worry as intensely as possible to test the prediction that it is possible to lose the mind due to intense worry. The experiment is preceded and then followed up with a very brief evaluation of the mental functions. For example: Are you still oriented to time, space and person? Do you still know your own social security number and your children's? Have you suddenly started to believe that you are being persecuted by foreign or domestic security services, or similar? Now, after the experiment: How much do you believe that it is dangerous to worry – between 0 (not at all) and 100 (completely convinced)?

If the danger meta-beliefs are mainly about worry or rumination leading to stress that damages the body, a similar experiment can be carried out where, for example, the client is asked to take a pulse or test blood pressure before and after an experiment where the worry is pushed to the maximum for a while. If the heart rate were to increase, which rarely happens, a continued dialogue could revolve around whether an increase in heart rate should be understood as an unhealthy event having occurred, or perhaps, on the contrary, a rather healthy one.

Interventions to challenge and modify fusion meta-beliefs

In Chapter 2, various fusion beliefs were described such as *thought action fusion* (TAF), *thought event fusion* (TEF) and *thought object fusion* (TOF). These beliefs are often evident in obsessive-compulsive disorder, but can also occur in other problems, such as health anxiety/hypochondria. Fusion beliefs are metacognitive beliefs that thoughts can influence actions, events, or objects in the external world. An example of TAF could be: "If I get an impulse that I suddenly push another person over in the city, the risk that I will do so increases". An example of TEF could be: "If I think of an accident, the probability increases that it will happen". Finally, an example of TOF could be: "I saw a photo of Adolf Hitler in an old book at home. What if Hitler's evil thoughts had been transferred to the book and now flow over to me every time I open or go near the book?".

Verbally, fusion beliefs can be challenged by asking the client for historical evidence and/or mechanism explanations. If the therapist asks for historical evidence to challenge thought action fusion (TAF), the questions could be, for example:

T: *How many times in your life have you had the impulse to commit a brutal act of violence?*
P: Oh, probably many thousands of times.
T: *How many times have you committed a brutal act of violence?*
P: Well, none.
T: *What does that say about the importance of those thoughts, do you think?*

If the therapist explores mechanism explanations together with the client, the dialogue could look like this:

T: *If you were to have an impulse to hurt someone even though you don't want to, what exactly would happen when you go from thought to action?*
P: I don't know if I can really answer that ...
T: *Doesn't it take anything more than a thought to carry out an action?*
P: What do you mean then?
T: *Yes, for example, an intention or a plan? If I get the idea that I'm going to London, will I automatically arrive in London?*
P: No, of course, not just by only thinking the thought. Of course, you both need to want to go there and do some preparation and planning for it to happen.

Already during the case formulation and socialization to the formulation, the client is made aware that he or she relates to certain thoughts as if they were very significant and powerful. For example, as if the thought that the iron at home is still on and hot increases the risk that it will soon start to burn in the client's home. Verbally, these types of beliefs are challenged through dialogues such as this one:

T: *You seem to appraise the intrusive thought of a switched-on electrical appliance at home as very important and powerful. Are all your thoughts powerful? For example, can you win at a lottery by thinking intensely about winning?*

P: No, I know it sounds a bit odd, but it doesn't apply to positive events.

T: *Why do you think it doesn't apply also to positive events?*

P: I don't know, maybe because those thoughts don't give me anxiety.

T: *But does it matter what you or I think about a turned-on iron? Or whether we have anxiety or not at the same time?*

P: Yes, I know it may sound illogical, but …

T: *Because either the iron is turned on even if we think it's off, or it's turned off and we think it might be turned on. Then, of course, it can be turned off and we think it's off or on and we also think it's on …*

P: Mmm.

T: *But can you turn your iron on or off at home with your thoughts? If so, how does it work? How much do you believe that your thoughts about a switched-on electrical appliance at home are important and can increase the risk of fire, on a scale between 0 and 100?*

Similar verbal challenges occur in thought action fusion (TAF). Note, however, that before further behavioral experiments to challenge TAF are carried out, it must have been clarified that obsessive thoughts about harming others are experienced as self-dystonic, self-alien to the client. People with OCD who have obsessive thoughts about harming others almost always answer that they would not want to turn the thought or impulse into action and that the action would very clearly be in opposition to their deep-rooted values and intentions. A verbal challenge of TAF in a client who at the same time describes the obsessive thoughts as ego dystonic can go like this:

T: *When you get the thought that you would suddenly abuse your own children sexually, you have told me that you usually get completely scared and almost panicked.*

P: Yes, I think those thoughts are absolutely disgusting and annoying. Those thoughts are just completely sick!

T: *May I ask, do you want to have sex with your children?*

P: Absolutely not. That's the last thing I want. That would be a despicable act.

T: *Why would you do that if you don't want to? Do you usually act on everything you think, or follow your every whim?*

P: Ehh … No, I probably don't.

T: *But coming to such actions you decide to carry out, like going to work, shopping for food in the store, going with the family on a holiday trip. Is it enough to get a thought in your head to get to work or go on holiday or do you also need something more? For example, motivation to do so, an intention, some planning and some preparation?*

Metacognitive behavioral experiments to challenge and modify fusion beliefs

Behavioral experiments can be used to challenge and modify fusion meta-beliefs regarding actions or events in the near future. One of these could look something like this:

T: *If it is the case that your thoughts are very important and have the capacity to harm others, can you try to hurt me with your thoughts?*

P: ?

T: *Can you give me a bruise here on the back of my hand by thinking intensely? Can you think as intensely as possible that you are giving me a bruise here with your thoughts?*

P: [After a minute or so] No, of course it didn't work. It's just that sometimes I don't dare to take the risk. If I get the idea that I may have hit someone with the car without noticing, it feels kind of dangerous not to be able to figure out what really happened.

T: *How much do you believe that the likelihood of hitting someone with your car increases if you were to have such an intrusive trigger thought?*

Experiments like the above can also be adjusted with thoughts of more serious harm. For example, the therapist could say, "Try to make me have a heart attack with your thoughts". The experiment can be followed up with a dialogue about whether the exercise has entailed any increased danger or not.

Additional behavioral experiments to challenge and modify fusion beliefs such as TAF, TEF, and TOF are described in Wells (2009).

Exposure with response prevention (ERP)

ERP can be used to challenge fusion beliefs or beliefs about rituals in OCD. Response or ritual prevention based on MCT means that the client in connection with exposure refrains from the ritual and all other CAS. CAS is to be understood as a response to the trigger. In MCT, the exposure is not used as extensively or as long as in CBT. In ERP, according to the MCT rationale, the client can, by refraining from responding to the obsession, discover that thoughts lack the meaning and power that was previously believed. When the client responds to and tries to neutralize the obsessive thoughts, the discovery that the thoughts themselves cannot influence external events or actions is prevented. For example, CAS prevents the discovery that it is something completely safe to have an impulse to harm someone else and leave that impulse without any kind of action or neutralization. During ERP, the client may be suggested, for example, to think intensely of themselves as contaminated and at the same time postpone their cleaning ritual. The purpose of the exposure is then not to get used to anxiety/habituate, but instead to be able to challenge the metacognitive belief (TEF) "if I have a thought of being contaminated and at the same time feel anxiety, it means that I am contaminated". After such exposure, a dialogue could follow about whether the client really believes that the thoughts and feelings have affected, for example, the bacterial content on the skin. The client could also be encouraged to think intensely about an accident that could occur and then be challenged in the belief that the probability of the accident occurring has changed in some way in connection with thinking about it. That is, exposure can be used to make it possible to discover that thoughts, impulses and emotions don't matter and can instead be regarded as temporary internal events, without the possibility of influencing external events. Likewise, ERP for OCD can be designed to challenge the meta-belief of a cleaning ritual as "the only way to be able to let go of the thought that I'm dirty, is by implementing my washing ritual".

Through exposure, the client can be helped to discover that the ritual works poorly to eliminate intrusive thoughts and that these will disappear by themselves after a while if the client applies DM. A meta-belief that the worries and obsessions will remain in the consciousness constantly if the ritual is not performed, can be challenged and modified. In ERP by the MCT rationale, the questions about the client's experience of anxiety do not become important in the way that they usually are in CBT. The direct goal is not to relieve anxiety, but to change meta-beliefs about, for example, the importance of thoughts. The MCT therapist may instead ask: "The fact that you feel anxious, does it affect the risk that you will commit a pedophilic act that you do not want to commit?" or "Can your feelings and thoughts affect how clean or dirty your hands are?" and further, "Would you still be afraid of your thoughts if you realized that they cannot make you do things you do not want to do and if you realized that they totally lack the importance you previously gave them?"

Exposure and response commission (ERC)

ERC can be used as an intervention/behavioral experiment in OCD. When carrying out ERC, the client is encouraged to perform their compulsive ritual, for example the usual cleansing ritual in connection with contamination thoughts, but at the same time keep the obsession in their consciousness. The rationale here is to increase the client's meta-cognitive awareness (it is thoughts, not dirt that is the problem), to reduce thought event fusion (TEF) (the thoughts say nothing important about how clean or dirty my hands are) or to reduce positive beliefs about the cleansing ritual. The rules change during the ERC, the obsession is kept in the consciousness throughout the ritual instead of trying to eliminate it from the mind. This is intended to make it easier for the client to switch the experience of intrusive thought from object mode to meta-cognitive mode.

Interventions to modify positive metacognitive beliefs

Interventions such as DM, postponement of worry and rumination, ATT and SAR can also be used to challenge and modify positive metacognitive beliefs. A person who has significantly reduced their worry may be asked by the therapist: "Have you done anything dangerous now? Has the reduced worry in any way increased the risks for you or your family? How much do you believe right now that worry protects you, helps you or makes you a better parent, on a scale between 0 and 100?" To a person who has radically reduced the time for rumination, a similar question can be asked: "Now you have hardly ruminated at all during the last week. Does this mean that the risk of relapsing into depression may have increased and that you have a poorer understanding of how to deal with your depression? Or is the opposite true? Have you missed something important by not ruminating? How much do you believe now that rumination will help you get out of your depression?" In a similar way, questions can be asked of a person with previous social anxiety and who now uses their attention externally in social situations instead of focusing on the negative image of themselves as a social object: "Do you handle the social situations worse now that you have stopped monitoring how you appear in the eyes of others?" or "How much do you now believe that worrying before social situations or rumination afterwards are helpful for you in your social life, on a scale between 0 and 100?"

In addition, positive metacognitive beliefs are also challenged and modified, both verbally and through metacognitive behavioral experiments. Verbally challenging can be done with questions such as:

T: *How do you know that you are worrying about the right things? If I go to myself, I can imagine several bad or catastrophic events that could occur only for the rest of this day. Maybe I'm worried about getting a falling icicle in my head when I go home and then I'll be hit by a drunk driver instead. Maybe I'll have a stroke. How do you know you're preparing for the right things?*

P: I often worry about different serious diseases that I don't want to have, but of course there are an infinite number of disasters that could happen …

Additional questions may be:

T: *Flying commercial flights with 300 passengers is probably not a completely risk-free business, or what do you think?*

P: No, if something happens, it usually gets very bad with many or all of them dead and mutilated.

T: *If you could influence it yourself and were responsible for their training, would you want the pilots to be risk-aware?*

P: Well, that's obvious.

T: *Do you want them to worry or just to follow their checklists and safety procedures?*

P: I would rather they concentrate on the safety procedures and handling of the aircraft than worry.

T: *How do you currently rate your belief that worry is important for reducing risks in life, on a scale of 0 to 100?*

To clients with health anxiety, the question can be asked: "On the last occasion when you met with your doctor, what information did you get? Were you really told that you can reduce your risk of cancer or heart attack by increasing your worry? How come you don't get a prescription for increased worry?" Should the client perceive the question as ironic and object: "I also understand that worry is not one of the risk factors for lung cancer, but I just can't help but worry", the dialogue goes back to challenging and modifying worry as uncontrollable.

Advantages and disadvantages analyses

If the client has residual positive beliefs about worry, rumination and other CAS, the therapist and client can jointly explore the potential advantages of CAS compared to the disadvantages and negative consequences. Above all, the pro/cons analysis becomes necessary if the client's positive beliefs about worry, and rumination becomes a blocker for continued therapeutic work to reduce repetitive negative thinking. Bearing in mind that CAS has so many negative consequences and that the client has sought help with their problem, the perceived benefits will usually be modest compared to the negative consequences. A client with OCD who controls the stove as a ritual, could still have some positive beliefs that this reduces the risk of fire, but then also must consider this perceived benefit compared to the vast negative consequences. A person with PTSD who isolates himself at home after an assault, could be encouraged to compare the advantages, such as the fact that the risk of a new robbery on a commuter train has now decreased to zero, with the disadvantages, such as that life still feels scary, restricted and anything but safe. A client with positive meta-beliefs about rumination could express advantages such as "Analyzing makes me a sophisticated and interesting person" and compare these with disadvantages such as "It is extremely rare that I enjoy social interaction when I ruminate. Besides, I never come up with anything that I didn't already know and my whole life usually feels uninteresting and meaningless when I've analyzed myself long enough".

Behavioral experiments to challenge and modify positive metacognitive beliefs

Metacognitive behavioral experiments that can be used to challenge positive meta-beliefs about worry or rumination are the mismatch strategy, and worry and rumination modulation (Wells, 2009). The mismatch strategy is used to examine the predictive value of worry. The client is then asked about things they have worried about earlier in life or are worried about now, and this is then compared with what the actual outcome has been or will be. For example, the therapist may ask:

T: *How many times have you worried that you might accidentally say something that makes others think you're odd and weird?*
P: I've worried about that since I was a teenager and for many years since then. Thousands of times at least.
T: *How often have people around you pointed out that what you say is odd and strange?*
P: Well, it has probably never happened.
T: *If you have worried thousands of times and it never happened, what does that say about the informational value/predictive value of your worry?*

The mismatch experiment can also be used prospectively. The client is then asked to describe a situation and portray in detail an outcome that they are worried about for the coming week. During the following session one week later, the therapist and client jointly examine how well the worry/ prediction and current outcome correspond.

In the case of remaining positive meta-beliefs, worry modulation can be used to explore the benefits of worry. For example, a client who has the idea that he functions better in his role and in his responsibility as a parent if he worries, can be encouraged to try days with worry and days without worry. The client can then try to worry as before treatment during the first two days after the session, and then practice DM and postpone worry the two days after that, and so on. During the next session, the experiment is evaluated, and new ratings of the positive meta-beliefs are asked for. It is likely that the client has also discovered other positive effects of reduced worry, perhaps that the relation with the children has improved. In the case of rumination problems, a similar experiment can be carried out.

Increased activity and interventions aimed at reducing avoidance and other CAS behaviors

Like other CAS elements, behaviors in case formulation are controlled by metacognition. Many behaviors, such as various forms of avoidance, alcohol use and safety behaviors such as reassurance seeking, turn out to be aimed at reducing and controlling worry or rumination. When worry and rumination come under control through the new alternative strategies, with the help of DM, worry postponement or ATT, the client feels that they have effective and alternative ways to reduce worry and to interrupt the negative persistent thought process. If one reason for social withdrawal has been to give yourself time and space to ruminate and you now have concluded that you neither want to ruminate nor need to do so, the motivation to isolate yourself usually will vanish. Various forms of social avoidance are often strategies to reduce worry. Once the client has discovered the ability to interrupt worry, the necessary step towards increasing activity becomes much easier to take. As well as worrying about a future social situation, having too little energy before or being drained of energy by social meetings, you can discover the opportunity to interrupt the worry and postpone it until later. If you also experience that social interaction can be enriching, fun, interesting and vitalizing if you turn your attention to other people and the external situation instead of spending time with your negative thoughts, another reason to isolate yourself falls. Those who used to worry about being negatively evaluated by others in social situations and who later discovered that the trigger thoughts are not important and that it is possible to stop worrying, usually find that the reasons for saying no to various social events have disappeared. A person who has previously used alcohol or other substances very intensely and from the metacognitive belief that "only by drinking myself unconscious can I get a break from the thoughts of how worthless I am", often has more options than the chemical substance to find relief from the thoughts. Anyone who has used distraction strategies in other ways such as staying in constant activity, having many temporary sex partners, binge eating or sleeping excessively can discover alternative ways of relating to negative thoughts.

One reason for reduced activity levels and social withdrawal may stem from beliefs of the importance of negative thoughts. "I can't get out of bed as long as it feels pointless, and when all these negative thoughts are occupying my mind" or "I can't go to the party if I don't feel motivated to or think it will be fun". In similar cases, avoidance and passivity become a way of waiting for and anticipating the disappearance of the negative thoughts, a strategy that will work poorly, and that will imply continued engagement with the thoughts, and which will also further reinforce the meta-belief of negative thoughts as important. Anyone who has instead discovered that the negative thoughts are both normal and unproblematic, and that it is possible not to respond to them, will have completely different possibilities. What I think about a coming activity doesn't have to be very important.

If low activity levels, avoidance and social isolation continue to persist despite radically reduced levels of worry and rumination, the therapeutic interventions will be directed towards problematic behaviors and avoidance. Therapist and client together explore the metacognitive beliefs behind these behavioral strategies and a plan will be developed for how an increase in activity can be achieved and how avoidances can be banned. Is there anything about an increase in activity that worries you? If so, how can you deal with those trigger thoughts? Do you cling to a view of yourself as incompetent or as doomed to fail? If so, are there any advantages to holding on to that belief of yourself as a failure? What will happen if you apply DM to similar thoughts? Are there any blocking beliefs that social activity leads to harmful stress and energy loss and that energy and vitality will be preserved by avoiding social gatherings? How well do similar beliefs match the client's previous life experiences? How can different metacognitive behavioral experiments be designed to test similar beliefs? A client who tries to save energy out of worries of otherwise becoming exhausted, could be given a homework assignment to try to overexert themselves with activities to see if exhaustion really occurs. What behaviors are important in the social situation in order to have the best possible conditions for a nice and positive exchange of time together? In general, the new rule "Don't think so much, just do it and try it out" is being tested. Therapist and client make plans, a so-called "new plan" for how the client should relate to trigger thoughts and use their attention, as well as for which behaviors seem more helpful than previous CAS activities.

Relapse prevention, new plans for processing

Prior to ending treatment, a plan is drawn up for how the client will continue to apply DM, interrupt and refrain from prolonged worry and rumination, use attention in more external and flexible ways, and continue with behaviors that will promote vitality and well-being. A special form is usually used for this purpose, *the new plan summary sheet* (Wells, 2009). In connection with metacognitive change, new "anti-CAS strategies" can be assumed to gradually feel more natural to engage in. If the client has discovered that worry and rumination are completely controllable processes regardless of external and internal events, the question can be asked: "Can something in the future happen that means that you no longer have that control?" Old habits are replaced by new ones. A life without persistent worry and rumination is experienced as liberating. You feel more alert, lighter, experience better concentration and find that interpersonal relationships work better and become more rewarding and stimulating. Often, so-called "booster sessions" are planned, where after a while you can follow up and find that the new plan can be adhered to and where you otherwise can remind yourself of and pick up on the new strategies that you developed during the treatment.

Therapeutic resistance, ambivalence towards change

The S-REF model provides new opportunities to understand therapeutic resistance in psychotherapy (Wells, 2019). Both positive and negative meta-beliefs control CAS, which means that an individual with generalized anxiety disorder may both experience their worry as very problematic and at the same time hold strong positive meta-beliefs about the worry as protective or helpful. A person with obsessive thoughts may find these very disturbing and at the same time have meta-beliefs about them as very important and too dangerous to ignore or apply DM to. Similarly, compulsive rituals are often experienced as both very painful and tiring to perform and at the same time dangerous to abstain from. A person with health anxiety may find the anxiety problems very bothersome and at the same time hold metacognitive beliefs that preoccupation with illness thoughts reduces the risk of becoming seriously ill. In PTSD, the client may have ideas that continued rumination is a way to get over the trauma or that continued worry protects their own mind. A person who is depressed may hold meta-beliefs that rumination is a way to heal and get out of depression. Uncontrollability beliefs or beliefs that the depressive thought processes are biologically controlled leads to pessimism and sometimes hopelessness, which may mean that the client imagines the therapeutic interventions as meaningless and therefore does not practice them as intended.

Furthermore, resistance in therapy can be about worries about possible loss of identity, risks of failing should they try the interventions, or new demands from the outside world. An individual who has identified herself as an anxious person after being a worrier all her life, may sometimes worry "What if I no longer know who I am without my worry? What if I become apathetic or emotionally cold then?" Anyone who suspects that a reduction in symptoms could lead to increased vitality and more energy, may sometimes worry that the progress will only be temporary and that any setbacks will mean that they are in a worse position than before the start of therapy. A person who holds on to thoughts of himself as being hopeless may worry about what it would feel like to fail after having worked hard and made a wholehearted effort to reach a goal. A person who has adapted to his thoughts of being unlovable may worry about how it would feel to have opened up, begun to hope for love and then be rejected. Furthermore, it is possible to worry, if you are getting better, that close relatives or other people around you will start to increase their demands and put faith in you and that you then will not feel ready to meet the new expectations. In MCT, similar worries are seen as new worry themes that are in no way significantly different from other worries. The S-REF model provides new opportunities to analyze resistance and motivational problems in therapy in terms of CAS and dysfunctional meta-beliefs, and thus also new opportunities to intervene against resistance using the therapeutic interventions and techniques described in this chapter.

5 Using MCT with common psychological problems, Part I

Anxiety and worry

Conceptualizing common psychological problems with the S-REF model

Based on the previous transdiagnostic discussion in the book, the categorization of mental health problems based on DSM and ICD can also be seen from another perspective, as superficial phenomena. Instead, the clinicians' focus can be on significant processes and mechanisms beyond the diagnoses and whether these can be made visible and modified in more effective ways. In MCT, the starting point is that CAS and dysfunctional metacognition constitute the central transdiagnostic processes that need to be targeted and influenced in psychotherapy.

In the upcoming review in this chapter and in Chapter 6, there are descriptions of CAS and metacognition also for the diagnoses GAD, PTSD, OCD and depression. For much more detailed and in-depth descriptions of these diagnoses, as well as of the treatment there, see Wells (2009). In addition, this chapter also describes the conceptualization of social phobia/social anxiety. Wells' contribution and the influences of the S-REF model are obvious in Clark and Wells' model of social phobia (Wells, 1997). This treatment has also been further developed and made more efficient based on a stronger anchoring in MCT (Nordahl et al., 2016).

Several disorders and emotional problems are highlighted in the following chapter and in Chapter 6. Should the review be perceived as long-winded and repetitive, it is of course possible to make a reference to selected sections on a particular disorder or a certain problem area that interests the reader. It should also be borne in mind that what constantly recurs are headings about CAS and metacognition, i.e. the underlying problematic transdiagnostic processes. Through this, the different DSM or ICD diagnoses can be seen as superficial phenomena. Seen from the perspective of the S-REF model, the psychological problems are significantly fewer than those listed in the following review.

CAS and metacognition in anxiety and worry problems

Worry is one of the central thought processes that is highlighted in MCT. Among the anxiety disorders it's particularly evident, but also in virtually all

DOI: 10.4324/9781003597100-6

psychological or psychiatric problems, it's possible to identify worry as a problematic maintenance process. Worry problems are thus found in many other problem areas than in those described below this heading. A diagnosis that is particularly characterized by worry problems is generalized anxiety disorder (GAD). In addition, worry is included as a central CAS process and as a diagnostic criterion for health anxiety/hypochondria and panic disorder.

Generalized anxiety disorder (GAD)

Hugo suffers phobias. Wasps, dogs, snakes, tight spaces, elevators, and heights are some of them. He has tried medications and various forms of psychotherapy. He has actually come to terms with the dog phobia after turning to a CBT psychologist and working actively with exposure to dogs, but several of the others remain. He becomes limited in his life, does not dare to travel to the countryside in the summer and thinks that he gets stuck in a negative social role as the one who always is afraid of all sorts of things. Hugo worries a lot about his elderly parents becoming seriously ill and dying, and he worries about his finances and that he may have chosen the wrong education. He also worries that all this worry might break him down and eventually cause him to lose his mind. A doctor at the health center has told him that, in addition to the phobias, he may also suffer from generalized anxiety disorder (GAD). And of course, Hugo thinks that the doctor is right in the sense that Hugo has always been a troubled soul and that he often feels tense and has difficulty relaxing. Another doctor as well as another psychologist has instead suggested that Hugo's problems may be rooted in an undiagnosed ADHD problem, which has made Hugo even more worried. Hugo often has a really hard time concentrating and he gets tired easily. He is worried that all the worry and anxiety will overload him and make him mentally ill.

CAS in GAD

In GAD, CAS manifests itself primarily as persistent worry, a worry that also results in enduring anxiety. The worry is perceived as both energy-consuming and difficult to control. For the diagnostic criteria for GAD to be met, several different worry themes must be present. If the worry revolves around only one problem, regarding possible health problems, the problem is rather classified as health anxiety or hypochondria. Those who suffer problems with generalized anxiety disorder are usually bothered by both so-called type 1 and type 2 worry. Type 1 worry is worry about negative life events that may occur. Common type 1 worries are usually about themes such as risks of one's own or loved ones' illness, accidents, disasters, finances, relationships, partner choice or career choice. How many major or minor disasters can occur in a person's life? Theoretically, of course, there is an infinite number of both desired and undesirable future scenarios. A person who worries a lot imagines the negative events above all and not so much the positive ones. That is, worry is thus a biased thought process towards threats and dangers. Even in moments that seem perfect, when everything feels nice in life, you can start to worry: "Is this too good to be true? Have I missed something? Do I challenge fate, do I invite a 'jinx' by relaxing and having a good time now?" The worry theme can be about the physical symptoms: "Now I have a lump in my stomach! Maybe it's my anxiety that creeps up again? What if it increases and makes me unable to function in the coming meeting at work?" Rumination can also occur: "Why do I feel so tense and anxious right now? Does that mean that I have missed paying attention to something important?" It is not uncommon for those seeking treatment for difficult to control worry to also start worrying that the treatment will not work or that they will have some kind of personal characteristics that mean that they are not receptive to treatment.

So-called type 2 worry, which also occurs in GAD, means that the person also worries about their worry: "What if I can't stop worrying and the worry never stops. What if the worry makes me sick? Maybe I can lose my mind from worrying? What if I get a stroke, cardiovascular problems, or even cancer from worry? What if I get fatigue, become burned out or completely apathetic from worry? What if the worry makes me unable to take care of my children or my other responsibilities in life? What if I pass my worries on to my children or if my partner gets tired of me because I always have to worry?"

In addition to the person with GAD devoting a lot of time and energy to worry, other typical CAS activity also occurs. Anyone who worries about possible illnesses typically scans the body and body sensations for symptoms. Anyone who worries about whether they currently live with the right partner often scans their feelings in an exaggerated way: "Do I feel any love right now? Do I feel anything at all?" Anyone who is worried about their children's health can scan for incipient symptoms of illness: "How is my child doing after the insect bite?" Anyone who worries about losing control of the bowel or bladder often scans for sensations from these areas of the body.

Typical CAS behaviors in GAD are to ask relatives for reassurance, for example: "Do you think this spot on my skin could be dangerous? Do you think my boss is disappointed in me?" Other behaviors can be Googling diseases. Using alcohol or PRN/ as needed medication to try to regulate anxiety is not uncommon in GAD. Many people try different forms of breathing techniques, but usually find that these are quite ineffective. Perhaps different healthy food preparations are tried with hopes that they will have calming effects on the entire organism? Some people try mindfulness meditation, but usually find that mindfulness does not provide effective relief from worry either. Physical exercise is usually a healthy habit, but exercise to reduce worry rarely works effectively. Another procedure to try can be self-compassion or various forms of positive affirmation, but even such strategies do not have any long-lasting effect on worry.

Various forms of avoidance occur, such as not daring to watch news on TV or films with themes that could make the worry activated and difficult to control. Anyone who thinks that worry is caused by overexertion and stress often tries to reduce their commitments and avoid high activity levels. That is usually not effective against worry and generalized anxiety, but rather reinforces a perception of an imminent threat and of one-self as a person who is fragile and vulnerable. In addition, there are typical mind control strategies, such as thought suppression: "No, don't think that the car your wife is in will crash!" or exaggerated reasoning: "What is the evidence that I may have a serious illness and what is the evidence against it?" Various distraction strategies are also common, such as distracting oneself with computer games, TV series or the like. Avoidance and other CAS behaviors often function as a form of secondary CAS, i.e. the purpose is usually to manage and reduce worry. For further descriptions of CAS and metacognition in GAD, see for example Wells (2009).

Metacognition in GAD

Negative metacognitive beliefs correlate with pathological worry; see for example Wells (2010). The diagnostic criteria according to DSM 5 and ICD 10 for the diagnosis of generalized anxiety disorder state that the worry should be perceived as difficult to control. This criterion corresponds to the negative metacognitive belief of uncontrollability. This negative metacognitive belief is what is most important to change during a treatment. The person who has later modified the belief of uncontrollability and through the treatment instead gained an experience of being able to control the worry and of being able to interrupt the worry process whenever they wish, usually feels that they have solved their previous problem in association to generalized anxiety. Another negative metacognitive belief in GAD is that worry is dangerous. It is common in GAD to think that too much worry can damage the body or mind. If the client has then undergone successful treatment with MCT and subsequently experiences the worry as completely optional, the possible problem with the worry as harmful usually disappears. If you think that the worry is harmful, but at the same time controllable, you probably choose to interrupt your worrying and to worry as rarely as possible.

Positive metacognitive beliefs also occur in GAD. Since worry is to be understood as a coping strategy, there are always beliefs of worry as vital, protective, helpful, etc. However, these beliefs are not always visible at a declarative, explicit level. It is not entirely uncommon for people with GAD to express themselves as "I see absolutely no benefits in worrying, only problems". Yet worry is conceptualized precisely as a coping strategy, albeit an unhelpful and counterproductive one. Positive meta-beliefs are also identified and challenged in MCT through the therapeutic dialogue and through various behavioral experiments. However, these are not assumed to be as important for the maintenance of the problem as the negative meta-cognitive beliefs. MCT in GAD, where the emphasis is on modification of metacognitive beliefs and reduction of CAS, has in comparative treatment studies outperformed the intolerance of uncertainty model (Af Winklerfelt Hammarberg et al., 2023; van der Heiden et al., 2012), Borkovec's avoidance model (Nordahl, Borkovec et al., 2018) and applied relaxation (Wells et al., 2010). Negative meta-beliefs have been shown to be more associated with the symptoms of GAD than, for example, intolerance to uncertainty (Penney et al., 2020). The metacognitive model has been shown to predict GAD and worry better than *the emotion dysregulation model* (Deleurme et al., 2022).

Health anxiety/hypochondria

Clinical presentations of health anxiety are in many ways like those of GAD. Diagnoses that according to ICD and DSM are best in line with the concept of health anxiety, is hypochondria according to ICD 10 and DSM-IV, and illness anxiety disorder according to DSM 5.

Tommy describes himself as a hypochondriac. "There is hardly any serious illness that I didn't think I had", he says. His friends are sometimes insensitive and make fun of him. They say that it shows on him when he starts to worry about a new disease. He looks worried and tense at these times, becomes short of words and quite absent. He gets the impulse to ask them for advice about his current symptoms, but refrains, guessing that he will be dismissed with something like "There is one disease that you suffer from and that is hypochondria!" The difficult thing, as Tommy sees it, is that you can never know for sure. He knows two people for whom a serious cancer diagnosis was discovered too late because they waited too long to contact the healthcare system, and others for whom serious diagnoses were missed by the doctor in charge. He has been to the health center quite a few times, but how do you know that the doctor is competent enough and interested enough to examine one? He quite often finds himself standing in front of the bathroom mirror, inspecting possible signs of illness in different parts of his body. As far as possible, Tommy avoids news reports about serious illnesses.

CAS in health anxiety/hypochondria

Worry, or preoccupation with fear about having or acquiring a serious illness or disease, is included in the diagnostic criteria for hypochondria/illness anxiety disorder. If the worry is limited only to this one theme of health and illness, the problem is referred to as health anxiety instead of GAD. Characteristic of health anxiety is a persistent worry about having or acquiring a serious illness. Of course, there are many medical conditions that seem both painful and devastating that you can worry about. It is not uncommon to worry about acquiring an illness that a family member or relative has been affected by or someone that has been noticed by the media. It is not unusual to worry about various types of cancer. A variant of health anxiety that occurs, but which is not as often described in the literature, is to worry about serious psychiatric conditions: "Am I losing my mind and my sense of reality? What if I can no longer distinguish imagination from objective reality?" Type 2 worry can also occur in health anxiety: "What if all this worry about illness will ultimately make me ill?"

Rumination in health anxiety is often about analyzing the origin of various symptoms. "When did this stomach discomfort really start? What could it have been caused by?" If this sounds like ordinary thoughts in connection with bodily ailments to the reader, one needs to keep in mind that rumination and CAS are characterized by persistent and repetitive negative thinking and biased attention.

Threat monitoring in health anxiety consists of internal scanning of body sensations associated with the symptoms, or external scanning of, for example, skin, redness, swelling, whites of the eyes. Typical CAS behaviors are asking relatives or health professionals for reassurance, excessively seeking contact with the health care system, reading a lot/Googling about diseases. Other behaviors can include checking the pulse and counting the heartbeat. Avoidance can appear as asking family members not to talk about illnesses because of easily aroused worries or not to contact the health care system at all at times when this would be recommended based on general health advice.

Metacognition in health anxiety/hypochondria

Like GAD, there are positive and negative meta-beliefs about worry and other CAS activity. Those who are bothered by health anxiety often hold positive meta-beliefs that worry about illness increases the chances of staying healthy, detecting illness in time or being prepared to deal with the emotional strain of contracting a serious illness. They will most often also believe that their worry about getting ill is uncontrollable. The experience is usually rather expressed as "I suffer from cancer worry" than "I choose to worry about cancer". Simultaneously with positive metacognitive beliefs about worry as lifesaving, there are negative meta-beliefs about worry as harmful, such as for example, that worry can cause cancer or serious cardiovascular disease.

Fusion meta-beliefs are prevalent and important to identify in the case formulation and treatment of obsessive-compulsive disorder (OCD), but fusion beliefs are also quite common in health anxiety. One fusion belief that quite often exists in health anxiety is *thought event fusion*, TEF. TEF means that the mere appearance in the mind of a trigger thought will be interpreted as if the probability of a negative event occurring thereby has changed. Examples of TEFs for health anxiety can be "if I get the thought that what I feel in my chest may be lung cancer, the risk increases that it is really lung cancer that I have acquired". Common ways to relate to a trigger about, for example, lung cancer, is to try to get rid of it through thought suppression, reassurance seeking, or by distraction. When the therapeutic dialogue has been switched from object mode to metacognitive mode, it becomes evident that similar strategies are aimed at controlling thoughts rather than the cancer risk per se. From a cancer perspective and with the aim of increasing a metacognitive perspective, one could continue to discuss "when it comes to the risk of lung cancer, can that risk be altered and changed by our thoughts?"

In a systematic review, including 36 studies, to examine the significance of metacognitive beliefs in health anxiety and somatic distress, Keen et al. (2022) found support for the S-REF model and for metacognitive beliefs as transdiagnostic factors. Bailey and Wells (2015) found that metacognitive beliefs moderate the effect between catastrophic interpretations and health anxiety, and in a later study (2016) that metacognitive beliefs predict health anxiety better than cognitive content in health-related catastrophic thoughts. Bailey and Wells (2014) also tested MCT in a case-series study and found that the S-REF model was applicable and that MCT preliminarily appears to be a promising treatment for health anxiety. Bailey and Wells (2024) conducted a pilot RCT with waitlist control (n = 20) and found MCT to be a feasible treatment with large effect sizes.

Panic disorder and other anxiety problems related to bodily functions, emotions and thoughts

It was terrible and so painful", says Viktor. I didn't understand what was happening to me and I thought I was about to collapse completely. It was as if everything just spun around. I was shaking and in a cold sweat. Later in the emergency room, the doctors found nothing wrong with me. They believed that I had experienced a panic attack. The first attack was not the only one unfortunately. I've been through it several times since then, and all this makes me very insecure. Today I can be afraid of trivial things like going shopping in the nearest grocery store.

Panic attacks are characterized by strong and sudden anxiety as well as physiological symptoms such as palpitations, pulse increase, sweating, dizziness, shortness of breath, chest tightness, nausea and numbness or tingling. The physiological symptoms are associated with a fear of dying or losing one's mind. People who have had panic attacks usually develop a so-called anticipatory anxiety for new attacks. It is also common to develop agoraphobia, i.e. fear and avoidance of, for example, public transport such as buses, trains and the metro, public spaces such as department stores, restaurants, theatres and cinemas. Agoraphobia (from the Greek *agora* meaning "market square") is not about "fear of squares" or fear of the public places themselves, but about the fear of having a panic attack in such a place. Panic disorder is something completely harmless. The usual catastrophe fantasies about dying or losing one's mind from anxiety are not realized.

Panic disorder is often described in terms of a misinterpretation of normal physiological sensations (Clark, 1986; Wells, 1997). In the case of strong fear, the physiological sensations that occur in a panic attack are amplified, which tends to be interpreted as evidence that something catastrophic is about to happen to one's own organism. Panic disorder is sometimes described as a phobic fear of one's own physiology. About 20 percent of the population is estimated to have had a panic attack at some point in their lives (Kessler et al., 2006).

Other anxiety problems related to loss of control of bodily functions

In other anxiety disorders, phobic fear and worry about interoceptive stimuli, inner experiences and one's own physiology also occur; see, for example, Boettcher et al. (2016). These include, for example, exaggerated fears of nausea and vomiting – emetophobia – (Boschen, 2007) or of losing control of bladder or bowel function (Kamboj et al., 2015; Pajak et al., 2013). Even with phobias such as flight phobia, height phobia or elevator phobia, it often turns out that the catastrophic fantasies/worries are related to something else or more than the risk of a plane crash, the high altitude itself or the fear of being trapped in an elevator. The catastrophic fantasies can instead revolve around losing control of oneself, one's body, emotions and one's own behavior. Fear of flying, for example, can be very similar to agoraphobia: "What if I have a panic attack inside the airplane cabin, lose my mind there and start behaving strangely?" (Wilhelm & Roth, 1997). A catastrophe fantasy in the case of a phobia of heights can be similar, but more fatal and stem from a fusion belief TAF: "What if I get an impulse to jump and at the same time lose control of my mind and my behavior?" (Hames et al., 2012). Similarly, the catastrophic fantasies in claustrophobia (Shafran et al., 1993), for example in elevator phobia, may revolve around fear and worry about one's own physiology and about loss of control over one's own emotions and behavior rather than about the elevator car crashing down the elevator shaft or for oxygen deprivation to occur in a stuck elevator.

CAS in panic disorder and other anxiety problems related to bodily functions

Worrying about new panic attacks and that they will lead to physical or mental damage is one of the diagnostic criteria for panic disorder. The worry in panic disorder can in several ways appear like that of GAD, although the anxiety experience in GAD is often more persistent, when instead the anxiety experience in panic is more sudden and short-lived. In both conditions, there is often worry about increased or continued anxiety, losing one's mind and losing control of one's own behavior. "What if anxiety makes me start talking weird or doing strange things?" What is described in panic disorder as anticipatory anxiety related to future panic attacks is merely to be understood as worry. "What if a new and even worse attack than the last one is on the way?" Otherwise, the worry can also revolve around the risk of social embarrassment and of having another panic attack in an inappropriate situation: "What if I have a panic attack in the middle of rush hour traffic on the subway? What if the subway train is full, I get stuck in a tunnel and I start to panic. What if I then start saying and doing strange things?" What was previously described as type 2 worry in GAD, i.e. worry about worry, seems very similar to catastrophic fantasies about losing one's mind and control over oneself and one's own mind. The presence of physiological sensations linked to fear is easily interpreted as evidence that a loss of control over mental functions is imminent.

Persistent and frequent worry about becoming nauseous or vomiting or no longer being able to control the bowel or bladder can by itself trigger and amplify sensations in the gastrointestinal tract or bladder. A person who is bothered by a phobia of elevators or flights can be free of worry for long periods of time, but if a situation arises where avoidance is no longer perceived as possible, the worry will be activated. People who are bothered by emetophobia/vomiting phobia can often say "it's not the moment when I vomit that scares me the most, rather the state before when I'm in uncertainty about whether the nausea will increase and whether I'm going to vomit or not". That is, such a statement can in a sense be understood as worry about the worry rather than about the vomiting itself. In addition to the worry described so far, it is not uncommon to also have social worry about the embarrassment of losing control of your body or behavior, and about what others will think about the chosen strategies for dealing with the worry problem. "What if others look down on me for not being able to travel by air?" or "Do they judge me or pity me for being an impaired and boring person who doesn't want to go to a theater performance or who can't relax and enjoy during a social event?"

Threat monitoring for those who worry about losing control of their anxiety, of their body's functions and of their behavior appears as scanning the pulse and heartbeat, the presence of any thoughts that might be appraised as strange, sensations of nausea, pressure in the bladder and pressure and movements in the gastrointestinal tract. Anyone who worries about losing touch with reality can scan experiences of unreality and in various ways try to check their mental functions to examine whether the perception of reality is still intact. If you worry about not being able to reach the toilet in time, you often get an overview of existing toilets nearby. A person who is worried about a flight can, in addition to scanning for unusual sounds and movements in the fuselage and engines, also scans for signs in facial features, tone of voice or body movements of the cabin crew that could signify that something is abnormal. In addition, there are body sensations, emotions and thoughts that could indicate incipient panic. A person who feels dizzy at high altitude can scan their symptoms of dizziness and anxiety, their perception of motor balance and possible impulses to take a step in the wrong direction.

CAS behaviors to deal with the problems described in this section consist of various forms of agoraphobic avoidance. Other behaviors include regulating worry and anxiety with medication, alcohol or other substances if necessary. Anyone who is worried about having a panic attack on the subway can sometimes complete the journey only together with their best friend or partner, but not on their own in rush hour traffic and preferably not through tunnels. When worried about losing control of the bowel or bladder, it is common to adopt a special diet or even avoid eating or drinking regularly, for example. Another behavior can be to go to the toilet a couple of times too often and "just in case". When worried about panic attacks, it happens that you avoid coffee completely for fear of triggering, for example, tremors and palpitations. It also happens that even small amounts of alcohol are completely avoided, not based on general health advice on the risks of alcohol, but based on worry that the physiology can be activated and that a loss of control of sanity and behavior may occur. Mind control strategies such as thought suppression or excessive planning of, for example, travel times and routes occur. A person who is afraid of vomiting can engage in excessive hygiene measures or ask relatives if they have washed their hands or if someone they have been with during the day has shown symptoms of nausea. Googling the search term "winter sickness" or similar is quite common among those who are preoccupied with the worry of vomiting.

Metacognition in panic disorder and other anxiety problems related to bodily functions

Metacognitive beliefs about the importance of controlling negative thoughts and emotions can occur, for example "in order to be able to ride the subway, I must not have any panic-related thoughts in my mind during the trip". The positive ones are about worry and other CAS activity as necessary and helpful coping strategies to prevent the catastrophe fantasies from being realized. Worry and threat monitoring are also perceived as difficult to control/uncontrollable. Worry is furthermore perceived as dangerous in the sense that it increases anxiety and symptoms and thus the perceived risk of new panic attacks, of increased nausea or of losing control of body, emotions or behavior. It is not entirely uncommon for fusion beliefs to occur, such as *thought event fusion* (TEF): "If I get the idea that I am going to pee on myself, the risk of it happening increases". *Thought action fusion* (TAF) also occurs, for example: "If I get the thought that I might start screaming loudly and uncontrollably out of sheer anxiety inside the airplane cabin, the risk that I will do so increases".

Cucchi et al. (2012) found an increased prevalence of negative metacognitive beliefs in patients with panic disorder compared to non-diagnosed individuals in a study that included 119 patients with panic disorder, 114 with OCD and 101 non-diagnostic participants. The patients with OCD also had an increased incidence of negative metacognitions. Aydin et al. (2019) similarly found an increased prevalence of dysfunctional metacognitive beliefs in patients with panic disorder and in patients with GAD compared to people without a diagnosis in a study that included 44 patients with panic disorder, 37 with GAD and 44 who were undiagnosed. Halaj et al. (2023) investigated clinical and cognitive insight among 83 patients who received internet-based CBT and concluded that, among other cognitive factors that are associated with insight, especially metacognitive beliefs are important in understanding awareness of symptoms and thoughts in panic disorder. Although it was a CBT treatment, dysfunctional metacognitive beliefs also decreased in the treatment.

While writing this, no treatment study of MCT specifically for panic disorder has been found. Johnson et al. (2017) conducted a randomized controlled trial where generic MCT was compared with CBT in mixed anxiety disorders, in 90 patients in in-patient care. The primary diagnoses in the patients were panic disorder with and without agoraphobia, social phobia and post-traumatic stress disorder – PTSD. The patients with panic disorder as their primary diagnosis were randomized between generic MCT and Clark's model for panic disorder. The patients with social phobia and PTSD as primary diagnoses and who were randomized to CBT were treated with the Clark and Wells model of social phobia (Clark & Wells, 1995; Wells, 1997) or Foa and colleagues' *prolonged exposure* for PTSD respectively (Foa et al., 2007). One conclusion of the study was that generic MCT provided faster treatment success for the patients in the study overall, but that the specific CBT treatments and generic MCT appeared to be equivalent at follow-up one year later. However, the authors highlighted the benefits of being able to treat different anxiety conditions with a generic treatment (MCT) instead of several separate CBT protocols.

Simons and Vloet (2018) conducted a case-series study of MCT with three adolescents with emetophobia, 14–17 years old, where they applied the generic MCT formulation for the treatment. The three patients recovered, and the authors concluded that MCT appears to be a meaningful explanatory model and treatment for emetophobia.

Social phobia/social anxiety

Karl usually finds it difficult to socialize and meet new people. He feels very tense in such situations, and he experiences the situations as him being expected to perform and being critically scrutinized and evaluated. In social situations, he tends to become very self-aware and cognizant of how his anxiety and social difficulties might become visible to others. As far as possible, he tries to avoid speaking during meetings at work, and often finds excuses not to go with his colleagues to lunch. Some social events are harder than others to avoid, such as family reunions or the company's annual Christmas dinner. On similar occasions, he may worry for days in advance. In addition, he can spend a lot of time afterwards thinking about how others perceive him. This type of post-analysis is often associated with anxiety and gloom, as well as an experience of being hopelessly apart, odd and lonely. He feels trapped in himself and wonders what is wrong with him, as one who experiences social interaction almost exclusively as a torment.

Social phobia or social anxiety is one of the most common anxiety problems. Social anxiety is about the worry of being negatively judged in encounters with other people; see for example Wells (1997). Most people have probably been through situations where they have experienced social anxiety. Instead of opportunities for joy and inspiration, social situations are portrayed in social anxiety as threatening and as occasions when negative evaluation of one's own person and one's own performance should take place. What is the intended performance about in case of social anxiety? The worry about performing poorly in front of others can be related to things such as not appearing intelligent and knowledgeable enough, sufficiently relaxed, "nice" and easy-going, funny, spiritual and so on. Some people find larger groups the most difficult: Situations like speaking or giving a lecture in front of a group, others may find it most difficult to, for example, have lunch with a colleague or their boss. Those who experience major difficulties also tend to develop secondary problems because of avoiding important opportunities for personal growth and the challenges and responsibilities that normally come with higher education, career and family life.

CAS in social anxiety

A person who is bothered by social anxiety worries about social situations and that others will perceive them as boring, unintelligent, stiff or weird. They also worry about getting anxious or not finding topics of conversation, or in various other ways not being able to handle the social situation. If you worry a lot in advance, you are often anxious already when you enter the social situation. Rumination is also a significant problematic CAS process in social anxiety. The rumination process is usually described here as "post-mortem", after death. That is, what you are engaged in is an exaggerated and repetitive analysis of social encounters that are already past and ended. Post-mortem rumination leads to a prolonged experience of anxiety, but also to a distorted negative view of one's own performance in social interactions; see for example Gavric et al. (2017).

When generating the case formulation of social anxiety, it makes sense to examine what happens before, during and after social situations. Social situations are preceded by worry and often also exaggerated planning of what to say and how to handle the social situation. Such planning usually complicates and perpetuates the perception of an imminent threat. After social situations, as already mentioned, post-mortem rumination occurs.

During social situations, a special form of threat monitoring usually occurs, an excessive checking of "self as a social object". "Self as a social object" refers to an imagined image of how the person looks and appears to others, i. e. a kind of imagined inner reflection of one's own appearance in social situations. The imagined image is negatively biased and fed by interoceptive data based on anxiety symptoms. If the individual feels hot in the face, it is easy to get an exaggerated image of themselves as red as a tomato. Alternatively, the inner image can be of the individual himself as corpse-pale, shaking like an aspen leaf, profusely sweating, etc. In MCT, "self as a social object" is conceptualized as a trigger thought, i.e. as a thought that the person with social anxiety over-engages in. CAS during an ongoing social interaction is usually about monitoring and efforts to control the imaginary and intrusive image "self as social object". It can be continuously monitoring how the heat in the face develops, how the tremors in the hands continue or how the sound of one's own voice sounds. It can also be to continuously review one's own conversational performance: "Oh no, why did I say that? It was a stupid thing to say!" Some of the symptoms of social anxiety are concentration problems and a feeling of being empty of thoughts. The explanation for these symptoms is that the person with social anxiety monitors, reviews and monitors themselves and at the same time tries to interact socially. All of this becomes an overly demanding and exhausting cognitive task. Anyone who interacts in this way appears to others easily absent, reserved and somehow uninterested. Sometimes monitoring also revolves around mind reading and trying to guess how others perceive their own person in the social situation or figuring out what the other person would prefer to talk about.

CAS behaviors tend to be performed with the intention of trying to hide and mask "self as a social object" from others. What can you do to hide your redness, tremors, and sweating? Is it possible to look a little more relaxed? What can you do to prevent others from perceiving you as boring, stiff or intellectual? Avoidance, i.e. declining or cancelling social invitations, is a common strategy. Other common safety behaviors are avoiding eye contact, dressing in a way that is thought to mask sweating, or keeping your hands close to your body to hide shaking. Sometimes it can also be about smiling a lot to try to convey goodwill, yawning to try to relax, talking quickly to try to distract oneself/push away trigger thoughts about "self as a social object" or asking many questions to try to turn the focus away from oneself.

Many people turn to alcohol when trying to get more relaxed during social interaction. Taking beta-blockers and other medications are other ways to try to reduce worry and anxiety in social situations.

Metacognition in social anxiety

Examples of positive meta-beliefs can be "If I plan carefully what I'm going to say, I'll handle the situation better and others won't perceive me as weird/unintelligent". Or, "If I try to imagine all the questions I might get, I will be better prepared". Positive meta-beliefs about rumination can be "If I analyze how I behaved in the social situation, I will improve my social skills and find it easier to relax". Examples of negative meta-beliefs can be "in order to cope with social situations, I need to feel safe and relaxed" (i.e. the presence of tension and negative thoughts about myself makes it impossible to interact socially). Worry, rumination and threat monitoring are at the same time experienced as difficult to control, as uncontrollable mental processes.

Nordahl et al. (2017) found that metacognitive change to a greater extent than cognitive change predicts symptom reduction in social phobia. Nordahl and Wells (2017) found that the metacognitive model, including meta-beliefs, explains the problems of social phobia better than traditional cognitive models. In addition, Nordahl, Nordahl et al. (2018) found that negative metacognitive beliefs predicted depressive symptoms in people with social anxiety.

Other anxieties related to appearance/apparition

Edith can't come to terms with her body. She finds various calluses around her stomach, back and thighs that she is disgusted by and sometimes experiences as "quivering dead fat". Edith knows that she is not really considered overweight according to general health advice. She still feels fat and feels it is a weakness in herself since she has not much control over her feelings of hunger and that she has not been able to get rid of her remaining body fat. Edith has devoted herself to countless diets over the years. Sometimes she has for a shorter period managed to lose weight, only to discover a few weeks later that she had fallen back into old eating patterns and gained her old weight again. She feels so lonely, lacking in character and sexually unattractive.

CAS in other anxiety problems related to appearance/apparition

In addition to social anxiety, in various forms of eating disorders and body dysmorphic disorder BDD, significant threat monitoring of, and worry and rumination about "self as a social object" can occur. CAS revolves around the imagined, biased and distorted image of appearance that the person believes others also perceive in the corresponding way and will find repulsive. In the case of eating disorders, worry and rumination are usually about losing control of weight and body shape, appearing fat in one's own eyes as well as in the eyes of others; see for example Fairburn (2008). Rumination and thought suppression in eating disorders have been shown to increase the tendency to binge eating (Smith et al., 2019), and rumination is also otherwise associated with eating disorders (Smith et al., 2018). In a meta-analysis, Palmieri et al. (2021b) found that repetitive negative thinking in the form of worry and rumination is a transdiagnostic process that is also involved in eating disorders such as anorexia, bulimia, and binge eating disorder. The authors believe that one of the clinical implications of the meta-analysis is that treatments that focus on reducing worry and rumination, such as MCT, should be considered in eating disorder problems.

The worry may revolve around the calorie content of upcoming meals or about others perceiving the person as fat. Furthermore, there is often an over-analysis afterwards, i.e. rumination about the calorie content of the last meal. The rumination can also take the form of self-accusations about lack of character and inability to put oneself above things such as hunger and thoughts of food. Threat monitoring can consist of excessively scanning one's own body, mirroring oneself or comparing parts of one's own body, such as the stomach, neck or thighs, with other people's corresponding body parts. It can be scanning for a feeling of bloated stomach. External monitoring in eating disorders is often to scan for possible calorie content in different foods before meals that are served.

Problematic behaviors in eating disorders include keeping a strict diet, avoiding regular and all-round eating, binge eating, inducing vomiting, using laxatives, or excessively exercising. The function of binge eating and vomiting seems to be to distract oneself from rumination and the negative affect associated with rumination (Selby et al., 2008). The likelihood of continued binge eating and vomiting also increases because of dietary restrictions and irregular eating.

In the case of body dysmorphic disorder, threat monitoring is also directed at "self as a social object", i.e. at the fantasized and biased image of one-self, which other people are also believed to perceive correspondingly. Even in this case, the imagined image, the trigger thought, is based on interoceptive data and on thoughts. Attempts by others to provide corrective information, such as "there is really nothing wrong with your appearance, on the contrary, I think you are cute, goodlooking" are usually futile and easily interpreted as expressions of pity or bad judgment. To some extent, threat monitoring is also aimed at mind-reading and trying to guess other people's real negative perceptions of one's own appearance. In addition, threat monitoring occurs such as checking in detail and for an extended time the imagined appearance defects in the mirror or making comparisons with body details of others, with other people's cheeks, noses, jaw areas, hair lines or lips.

The worry revolves around future situations when someone else will be disgusted by their own appearance and in the longer term about having to be excluded from possible love relations or from other social relations. The rumination resembles the post-mortem to social phobia: "How disgusted were they by my appearance? What were they really thinking?" A lot of persistent and repetitive thinking is also devoted to the theme of appearance correction, thoughts about improving appearance, and to ruminating about various surgical procedures such as remodeling the nose, lips, breasts or buttocks. In a similar way to social anxiety and eating disorders, it seems that one's own perception is distorted by rumination and by persistent, repetitive inspection and troubleshooting in front of the mirror.

Common CAS behaviors are isolation, avoidance of social situations, of eye contact where the face is exposed, or avoidance by turning away the part of the face that is imagined to be defective. Sometimes the person avoids looking at herself in the mirror, or uses makeup to try to hide parts of the face. Unfortunately, there is also an entire industry of plastic surgery procedures where people with body dysmorphic disorder risk being exploited and harmed. Much of the worry, rumination and other CAS may also be directed towards surgical procedures that have already been carried out.

Metacognition in other anxiety problems related to appearance/apparition

The problems described above will mostly be experienced from object mode, i.e. the person will relate to thoughts of defective appearance or grotesque body shape as to facts. Often there is a lack of metacognitive awareness that these are thoughts, thoughts that have been processed intensively during considerable time. In this way, it can be assumed that fusion meta-beliefs will be present, and *thought event fusion* (TEF). "If I have thoughts of myself as ugly, disgusting or fat in the eyes of others, it means that this is also the case".

Examples of positive meta-beliefs are that worry, rumination and threat monitoring will increase their own security by making the person more prepared for others' possible rejection and feared reactions of disgust. At the same time, the worry, rumination and the threat monitoring are perceived as difficult to control or uncontrollable.

Olstad et al. (2015) compared, by using the Metacognitions Questionnaire-30 (MCQ-30), dysfunctional metacognitive beliefs in a clinical group of 53 women with ongoing eating disorders with three control groups. The control groups consisted of 47 women with a self-reported history of eating disorders and psychiatric problems, 37 women with a self-reported history of other psychiatric problems and 66 women who reported no ongoing or previous eating disorder or psychiatric problems. The clinical group with eating disorders and the group with self-reported history of eating disorders showed significantly higher levels of dysfunctional metacognition compared to the groups without current or previous eating disorders. High levels of dysfunctional metacognition correlated positively with high levels of eating disorder symptoms. The strongest correlation was between eating disorder symptoms and the subscale of MCQ-30, "Need to control thoughts", which includes, for example, the statement "Not being able to control my thoughts is a sign of weakness". The authors believe that eating disorder problems can be understood as maladaptive coping strategies to control worry and rumination. Furthermore, they believe that the results further underline the importance of dysfunctional metacognitive beliefs as transdiagnostic factors, not only in other problems, but also in eating disorders. Palmieri et al. (2021a) also found, in a systematic review that included eleven studies, a clear association between eating disorders and dysfunctional metacognition.

At an outpatient clinic for eating disorders, Lawson et al. (2022) tested modified MCT, i.e. MCT in combination with regular eating disorder interventions for anorexia (the regular eating disorder interventions were psychoeducation about eating, setting eating goals and regular weighing). The sample included 24 clients with anorexia diagnosis, of whom 12 completed the program/could be followed up with post-measurements. Eating disorder symptoms, depressive symptoms, worry/rumination, and metacognitive beliefs decreased significantly among clients who completed. The authors concluded that the modified MCT appears possible to be used successfully with this patient group and that larger controlled studies should be conducted. Robertson and Strodl (2020) conducted a small case series study of three clients with binge eating disorder where the conclusion was that MCT seems to be a promising model for the client group and that none of the clients met the diagnostic criteria by the end of treatment.

Anxiety – or worry disorders?

Many of the problems that clients seek help with are referred to in the diagnostic systems as "anxiety disorders". These include disorders such as generalized anxiety disorder (GAD), panic disorder with or without agoraphobia, health anxiety/hypochondria, social phobia or social anxiety, post-traumatic stress disorder (PTSD), obsessive-compulsive disorder (OCD) (previously according to DSM-IV), specific phobias such as a phobia of snakes, insects, dogs, etc. In addition to these anxiety disorders, anxiety as a problem also occurs in most other emotional and psychiatric problems, such as in depression, in personality disorders such as borderline personality disorder or emotionally unstable personality disorder, in psychotic disorders and in various forms of addiction/substance abuse.

In addition, it is not uncommon for people to seek psychological treatment for problems such as performance anxiety, test anxiety, claustrophobia, fear of flying, fear of vomiting and sometimes – and even though it never usually happens – of not being able to control the bowel or bladder. Among children, there is separation anxiety and an exaggerated fear that their parents will disappear. Sometimes even eleven-year-olds do not dare to sleep away from home or go on camps or school trips. In other cases, social anxiety and other fears, such as fear of the dark, occur in children. In all the problems mentioned above, it is evident that the individual worries a lot.

Based on the S-REF model and MCT, it could be questioned whether "anxiety disorders" or "anxiety problems" are really accurate concepts. For example, in the case of generalized anxiety disorder (GAD), one of the most common disorders among patients seeking help for psychological and psychiatric problems, the core problem is usually worry. One of the basic criteria for the disorder is persistent and difficult-to-control worry. Based on MCT, CAS is the activity that creates and maintains psychological problems, and anxiety is understood as one of the consequences of CAS. That is, the person who intensely and repeatedly worries and persistently tries to predict small and large disasters, will as a result experience more fear and anxiety. Sometimes this anxiety seems to be taken as evidence that there are good reasons to worry, that is, there is then a mutual connection between anxiety and worry, for example: "Why do I feel anxious right now? What's wrong? What is it that my unconscious is trying to tell me? Have I missed something important?"

Both pharmacological and psychological treatments for GAD, where the treatment targets are rather to relieve anxiety than to directly and specifically intervene against the worry process, seem not to be very effective. The prediction that can be made from MCT is that if you find new strategies that give genuine experience of being able to control the worry, the previous problems with anxiety will thereby disappear.

In clinical practice, panic attacks are regarded as completely harmless. Still, when experienced as very scary and problematic by the individual, the person often tries to deal with the panic in various ways and tends to approach it as if it was an immediate threat to their mental or physical health. The best advice to those who are bothered by panic disorder is often "do nothing, just continue with what you were doing". It is common to develop so-called anticipatory anxiety after a first attack. Since many somatic sensations such as palpitations, shortness of breath, tremors, dizziness, sweating and some cognitive symptoms, such as feelings of unreality, occur in panic attacks, anticipatory anxiety usually involves being extra-vigilant for just such symptoms. It is also very common to develop agoraphobic avoidance. Not primarily because such situations or places are suddenly now perceived as frightening in themselves, but because the person is worrying about having new panic attacks in similar situations. In MCT, agoraphobic avoidance and other avoidance can usually be understood as strategies to reduce worry. By avoiding, for example, public means of communication, the worry about a panic attack on the bus will be reduced.

A more accurate and useful term than anticipatory anxiety or agoraphobic anxiety is probably worry. Worry is thinking about bad things that may happen in the future, and the content of the worry theme is not important. Given that there seems to be an effective and general cure for all worry regardless of the content of the thoughts, it may make more sense to talk about worry problems rather than anxiety problems. Whether the fear revolves around having another panic attack and that it will be worse than the previous one, or whether one feels anxiety when thinking that the next panic attack might come inconveniently in a crowded subway car or in a theater, this could be defined as worry.

6 Using MCT with common psychological problems, Part II

PTSD, OCD, depression, sleep problems, prolonged grief and more

Post-traumatic stress disorder (PTSD)

After the car accident six months ago, Britta no longer feels like the same person. Physically, she is starting to recover, but not mentally. She almost never sleeps a whole night, is tormented by nightmares and is on edge most of the time. She has become anxious, bitter and depressed. Even though she has survived, she has begun to think that it would be easiest to just end her life. So far, when it's a possible option, she avoids going out because her anxiety is triggered both by moving cars and crowded streets in the city. She no longer drives, nor does she travel as a passenger. On occasions when she still has to leave her flat, she now always keeps a close eye on vehicles moving towards her or moving in her vicinity. She jerks slightly at sudden traffic noises. Britta has begun to wonder if her mind and brain has changed forever. Maybe her brain has been damaged by all the anxiety and stress. She feels like she's in a bubble, trapped in herself and is rarely emotionally touched as before. She has started to drink more often than before but has also noticed that this makes her situation even worse. She worries about the nightmares she still has and that her condition will deteriorate further. Britta has tried repeatedly to remember the exact sequence of events before the accident, her own actions and choices second by second. She is horrified at not being able to reach complete clarity in her memory fragments.

After traumatic events such as war experiences, torture, natural disasters, accidents, assault, or sexual abuse, some people develop symptoms like those of PTSD. The nature of the trauma, the severity and duration as well as the availability of social support are factors that are considered to play a role, as well as the presence of other psychological problems. The symptoms are characterized by re-living/flashbacks and recurring nightmares about the trauma event, by avoidance of places, people, activities, feelings and thoughts, by altered arousal reactions such as anxiety, irritability, hypervigilance and difficulty falling asleep, and by experiences of being alienated from others and of being changed as a person. According to SBU, (Swedish Agency for Health Technology Assessment and Assessment of Social Services), SBU (2020), about 25 percent of those who have been exposed to

DOI: 10.4324/9781003597100-7

traumatic events later develop PTSD, but this proportion varies depending on the type of traumatic event. For example, the proportion increases to up to 50 percent after experiences of torture and rape.

Most psychological treatments developed for PTSD include elements of exposure to trauma memories/processing of the trauma memory. Often, such steps are considered necessary. In MCT, the development of symptoms after traumatic events is explained in a different way and no exposure to memories or processing of trauma memories is needed according to the model.

CAS *in PTSD*

As with other problems, the development of symptoms into PTSD is explained by CAS and by the metacognitive beliefs that control the CAS. Many of the symptoms, such as increased vigilance, reliving, nightmares and anxiety, are considered natural reactions after a traumatic event and as part of a normal and temporary adjustment process. However, due to CAS, symptoms become persistent or even worsen. Some of the diagnostic criteria according to DSM 5, such as various avoidances, are according to the metacognitive model to be conceptualized as CAS behaviors, i.e. as coping strategies and thus not symptoms. Experiences of being changed and alienated, even sometimes experiences of "having broken down", are to be conceptualized as consequences of CAS, as products of rumination, worry and long-term internally focused threat monitoring. Both worry and rumination occur as problematic thought processes in PTSD. The worry concerns both the risk of new traumatic events, new abuse or accidents occurring and the symptoms themselves: "What is happening to me? What if I never will be the same and be able to function normally again? Am I getting worse?" A special form of rumination, so-called *gap-filling*, occurs. Gap-filling is to return to the memories of the trauma repeatedly and to try to fill memory gaps. "Do I remember every sequence of the trauma event? What happened just before that moment? What did I do next?" Positive meta-beliefs about gap-filling may be that you need to remember every moment of a trauma event to come to clarity about guilt and responsibility issues or whether something could have been done differently. Just like other CAS, gap-filling leads to maintenance of anxiety, insecurity and an ongoing engagement in memories of the trauma event. Another problematic consequence is that, since it is not realistic to be able to remember every moment of an event, you will become increasingly concerned about your cognitive capacity and your lack of memory. In addition to gap-filling, there is also other self-punishing rumination in the form of self-accusations for what has happened. Threat monitoring is directed both externally and internally in PTSD. For example, checking out for threatening people or other stimuli in the environment that reminds you of the trauma, such as sudden footsteps behind you, is common.

The problem with this external threat monitoring is, of course, that there are an unlimited number of potential threats to keep an eye on in the environment, and it becomes difficult or even impossible to relax. Internal threat monitoring also occurs, directed at the symptoms and at experiences of having been changed forever and having one's mind or brain damaged.

CAS behaviors in PTSD consist of various forms of avoidance of places, situations, people, thoughts and feelings. Thought suppression occurs as a significant and problematic process. Trying to suppress thoughts, memories and dreams makes them more frequent and intense, which is easily interpreted as the person's mind and brain being damaged. It is also common to try to self-medicate with alcohol or other substances to reduce the occurrence of intrusive memories and trigger thoughts or to try to decrease worry and rumination. Espeleta et al. (2021) showed that among people who develop PTSD after childhood experiences of neglect, repetitive negative thinking (RNT) and a low degree of attentional control had a significant influence on symptom development.

Metacognition in PTSD

As already mentioned, the CAS is controlled by, among other meta-beliefs, positive beliefs that worry, rumination and threat monitoring will reduce the risk and increase preparedness for new traumas. Other positive meta-beliefs are that the trauma must not be forgotten because continued processing of it is the only way to get over the trauma and to be able to move on in life. Further positive meta-beliefs controlling continued rumination can be that the person will thus become clear about responsibility issues and who is to blame for the traumatic event. Negative metacognitive meta-beliefs concern, among others, the meaning of the symptoms and the danger associated with them, such as beliefs that intrusive memories, dreams or anxiety can degenerate the mind and brain and lead to mental collapse. The symptoms and the presence of intrusive memories can be perceived as signs that the brain has been damaged, that one is a weak character/person or that deep down inside one has had a desire to be traumatized. Much of the worry, rumination and threat monitoring are perceived as difficult to control or uncontrollable.

MCT has been compared with *prolonged exposure* (PE) in PTSD (Wells et al., 2015), with *eye movement desensitization and reprocessing* (EMDR) (Nordahl, 2016), and with exposure-based treatments as *treatment as usual* (TAU) (Nordahl et al., 2024), and in these studies, MCT has surpassed EMDR, TAU and shown at least as good results as PE. The benefits of a treatment that doesn't include exposure to or the processing of traumatic memories are of course obvious.

Obsessive-compulsive disorder (OCD)

Obsessive-compulsive disorder is characterized by both compulsions/rituals and obsessive thoughts, where the compulsions are conceptualized as strategies to deal with the obsessive thoughts, neutralize them and thus reduce stress and anxiety. Sometimes there are only obsessions without compulsions. Obsessions are intrusive and unwanted thoughts, inner images or impulses associated with anxiety and discomfort. Not infrequently, the obsessions have content of a taboo nature, about violence, sex or religion. At other times, the thoughts may revolve around doubts about whether, for example, you have locked the front door at home, turned off the stove and other electrical appliances or if you are clean enough on your hands or around your intimate hygiene. We all have these kinds of thoughts, but the person who suffers from obsessive-compulsive disorder seems to relate to them in a different way, perceiving them as more significant, important and dangerous. That is, the problem is in an obvious way a metacognitive problem.

Frida is bothered by obsessive thoughts. They are unpleasant and scary thoughts that she has accidentally seriously hurt other people or that she could start behaving in an uncontrolled and weird way. She emphasizes that she never behaves aggressively or recklessly and that she is rather perceived as a kind, caring and very empathetic person. She also has some other time-consuming rituals such as checking whether the stove and electrical appliances at home are turned off before she leaves home and whether the door is properly locked. Similar rituals can periodically become quite time-consuming, and Frida feels stressed when she is performing them. Frida has tried both medication and CBT, with exposure and response prevention, to come to terms with the obsessive-compulsive problems. "Yes, of course the treatments have been partly helpful", says Frida, "but at the same time I'm sitting here in your office and I'm far from recovering from the problems". In addition to the fact that her obsessive-compulsive problems are very time-consuming and tiresome to engage in, and in addition to the fact that they cause a lot of anxiety in everyday life, Frida describes problems with cognitive confidence. "It's like I can't trust my five senses, my own memory and my own abilities to reason properly", she says.

CAS in OCD

Compulsive rituals are conceptualized as CAS behaviors and as responses to triggers/obsessions. The rituals also constitute attempts to regulate worry or rumination. "If I don't keep washing my hands, my worry will persist". Thought suppression is a highly significant process in OCD. A very large part of the worry, rumination, threat monitoring and the compulsions/rituals are driven by a wish to erase the obsession/trigger from consciousness. For example, repeatedly checking whether the stove is turned off or whether the front door is locked can be conceptualized as a desire to eliminate the doubt from consciousness, "to be done with it". However, both thought suppression and other CAS will have the opposite effect, i.e. lead to increased frequency of obsessive thoughts and a heightened perception of the thoughts as important and harmful. Some compulsions are covert rituals enacted to neutralize the obsession, such as counting, saying prayers or silently, for oneself, pronouncing affirmations. In addition to external and internal compulsive rituals, asking for reassurance is also common, such as:

"Do you think I may have said something inappropriate to this person I met yesterday?" or "Do you think I can infect my children with asbestos if I walk past a house with fibre cement at fairly close range and then give them a hug?" (The latter obsession sounds absurd, but that is how absurd the OCD logic can often be, even if the person otherwise shows a high intellectual and good social function.) Avoidance also occurs. A person who is preoccupied with worries about contamination sometimes establishes different cleanliness zones in the home and can avoid inviting his own friends over or allowing friends of his own children to visit. Sometimes your own cleanliness rituals can be perceived as so time-consuming, complicated and tiresome that you simply give up and stop taking care of your daily hygiene.

In OCD, a lot of time and energy is spent on worry and/or rumination. If the obsessive thoughts are related to contamination/dirt, the worry revolves around being soiled or dirty, despite the completion of cleaning. The worry can also revolve around the risk of accidentally infecting others. Sometimes obsessive thoughts and worry are related to the theme of hurting others. "What if I suddenly have an aggressive impulse and – even though this is something I really don't want to do – carry out an act of violence against a person around me or against a family member? What if I've already hurt someone or said something highly inappropriate without noticing it or remembering it?" Obsessive thoughts, worry and rumination may also be related to things such as forgetting to lock the front door, turning off the stove or other electrical appliances, turning off water taps and the like. "What if my mind deceived me and the front door is still unlocked?" or "What if I cause a fire at home by forgetting to turn the coffee maker off?" Although compulsive rituals, such as repeatedly checking that the front door still is locked, are intended to dispel doubtful thoughts, they instead have the opposite effect. No matter how many times you check something, there is always room for more doubt. Maybe your perception or memory deceives you? Anyone who has obsessive thoughts about electrical appliances sometimes deals with these by photographing the switched off stove controls before leaving home, but can you be one hundred percent sure that it is the most recent photo you are looking at if you then check to be certain?

Further worry and rumination may revolve around the meaning of obsessive thinking. "What does it mean that I get these kinds of impulses? Is it because I'm a latent sex offender? Does that mean that deep down inside I want to have sex with children? Does it even mean that I've had sex with children even if I don't remember it? Maybe I've even repressed the fact that I did it?"

A form of gap-filling rumination or scanning of memory images also occurs in OCD. "How did it really feel when I stood there and locked the front door? Did I hear that it clicked as it should?" If the theme of obsessive thoughts revolves around violence or accidentally hurting others, the rumination may consist of going back to memories of, for example, the last car ride: "Do I remember every moment of the journey? Was I inattentive at any point? Could it have been a blow to the car, or something soft I drove over without really noticing?" Since most of us do not possess such memory capacity, the results of the memory scan will be frustrating – there are always gaps in the memory. Often in OCD, this is not interpreted as a natural and completely normal limitation of human memory capacity, but instead it leads to a lack of confidence in one's own memory capacity and furthermore also a lack of confidence in one's own level of knowledge and in one's own senses. Gap-filling rumination, repeated control rituals and other CAS in OCD gradually lead to a growing doubt about one's own mental ability: "Am I seeing correctly? Can I trust my perceptions? Do I remember correctly? Can I trust my own judgment?"

External threat monitoring of, for example, dirt or remnants of bodily secretions, occurs in the event of obsessive thoughts related to the theme of contamination. At other times there is checking of controls, buttons and electrical contacts on electrical appliances. Internal monitoring also occurs, for example in the form of vigilance against taboo thoughts, or feelings such as: "Are there signs of sexual attraction somewhere in my body for this person? For this person about whom it would be completely disgusting and morally reprehensible to feel excitement?" In the case of obsessive thoughts that the front door has not been locked or the stove turned off, it is also common for so-called interoceptive data (i.e. feelings and body sensations) to be perceived as important. "What was my gut feeling when I locked the door the last time or when I looked at the stove buttons? Did it feel right?" Similarly, after a cleansing ritual, someone who has obsessive thoughts about contamination can scan off: "Do I feel clean now?" In general, monitoring of emotions can become very prominent and based on notions that fatal wrongdoings can be committed or even may have been committed with a clouded mind, and if the person does not feel perfectly alert, rested and sharp. That is, worry, rumination and threat monitoring can also revolve around the theme "Am I/was I sufficiently awake, concentrated and attentive?"

Object mode and metacognitive mode in OCD

In OCD, the experience tends to be very much in the object mode. The person suffering from OCD behaves in a way as if the problem was about contamination, hygiene, the risk of hurting others or the risk of really leaving the stove turned on or the front door unlocked. The metacognitive explorative dialogue aims to make the client aware that the problem is metacognitive. The dialogue needs to be switched to a conversation about thoughts and the way the client relates to thoughts. The therapeutic conversation for OCD is not about the risk of fire, forgotten stovetops, unlocked front doors, hygiene, risk of infection, risks of inadvertently harming others, but about thoughts about all this and how the person relates to these thoughts. It is precisely this systematic and consistent shifting of the dialogue from object mode to metacognitive mode that can be experienced as particularly challenging for the psychologist/ psychotherapist working with OCD problems.

Metacognition in OCD, fusion beliefs –TAF, TEF, TOF

Different forms of fusion beliefs occur in OCD, i.e. beliefs about the obsession/trigger thought as particularly important, powerful and potent enough to change the risks of various forms of disasters or unwanted events in the external world. *Thought action fusion* (TAF) means that a person who has an obsessive thought about harming a loved one believes that this intrusive thought increases the risk that the person will also act on that thought or impulse. (In dialogues with people who are bothered by thoughts of harming others, it is of course important to assess if this is a thought/impulse that the person would like to act on or if the impulse is ego dystonic. People with OCD describe obsessions about accidentally hurting others as definitely ego dystonic and completely against their deeply rooted values and desires, and thus similar obsessions will be considered completely harmless. Should the person instead describe the thoughts of harming others as ego syntonic and in line with what the person wants to carry out, risk and danger assessments will of course be needed and the continued clinical procedures will instead follow clinical guidelines for risk management, thus different from MCT for OCD.) *Thought event fusion* (TEF) is a belief that the presence of an intrusive thought affects the risk that something undesirable in the external world has already happened or will occur. "If I think that I have feces on my hands, it increases the likelihood that they are not clean". Or "If I think that my partner is going to crash the car this evening, the risk that it will really happen increases".

Another form of thought fusion sometimes occurs in OCD: *Thought object fusion* (TOF). TOF is a belief that negative thoughts and feelings can be spread to objects in the environment. For example, it may be objects that in some way through thoughts and feelings have been associated with bad luck, accidents or evil, and that these objects have now become infected and in themselves become unlucky or transmitters of misfortune or evil.

The fusion beliefs, which mean that the obsessions are perceived as important and dangerous, cause considerable anxiety in the person who is bothered by OCD. If the thoughts are perceived as dangerous, it is understandable that the person with OCD is also trying to deal with the thoughts and to neutralize them. "I can't shake someone's hand as long as I have a thought that there are feces on my hands" or "I need to think positive thoughts to prevent accidents and not being the one who causes a car crash". In TOF, the behavioral response can be to throw away objects and personal belongings, such as certain clothing that is associated with bad luck.

Further metacognitive beliefs in OCD

In addition to fusion beliefs, there are also positive and negative metacognitive beliefs about worry, rumination, and compulsive rituals. Beliefs about rituals are predominantly positive and related to rituals as necessary and even life-saving responses. "Just ignoring the thought and not performing the ritual could risk the lives of other people or myself causing a fire in the property where I live". "Trying to remember one more time will help eliminate the doubts about whether or not I have accidently watched child pornography". Other beliefs about rituals may be that the rituals will provide peace of mind and reduce worry and anxiety, for example: "If I didn't perform my cleansing ritual, I would worry for the rest of the day and not be able to attend to my list of tasks". In addition, in OCD, start and stop signals for rituals will be explored. An explorative question in the treatment of OCD can be "How do you know and decide that you are done with your ritual?" Common answers from the client are that the start and stop signals for the ritual are usually based on interoceptive data. "I check the door lock until it feels right and the feeling that I'm checking for is somewhere in my stomach or in my chest". A person with obsessive thoughts about pedophilia might answer, "I try to go through my memories until the doubt has disappeared and the anxiety has decreased".

Solem et al. (2009) found that metacognitive beliefs that changed during OCD treatment with exposure and response prevention predicted treatment outcomes better than changed cognitions. Sassaroli et al. (2015) investigated the association between OCD symptoms and the cognitive factor of inflated responsibility in 37 people with OCD and 31 people in the control group. They found that a correlation between inflated responsibility and symptoms existed, but that this was entirely mediated by negative metacognitive beliefs. In a study of 156 individuals from a non-clinical group, Gutierrez et al. (2020) found an association between anxiety sensitivity and OCD symptoms, and that the association was better mediated by metacognition than by *state/trait anxiety*. Kim et al. (2021) found among 562 OCD patients, compared to a control group without OCD, increased ratings of dysfunctional metacognitive beliefs. The authors interpreted the results as meaning that dysfunctional metacognition seems to play a crucial role in OCD. Hansmeier et al. (2021) found in a comparative study between MCT and ERP in OCD that altered start and stop signals in both treatments predicted reduced OCD problems regardless of treatment. Several studies, some of them RCTs with active control conditions, indicate that MCT appears to be an effective treatment for OCD (Carter et al., 2022a; Exner et al., 2024; Glombiewski et al., 2021; Melchior et al., 2023; Papageorgiou et al., 2018; van der Heiden et al., 2016). MCT has also been studied in pediatric OCD with encouraging results and large effect sizes. Reinholdt-Dunne et al. (2024) carried out a pilot study of group MCT with eight sessions with 11 pediatric clients and two 60-minute workshops for parents. The response and remission rates were 82% and 55%, respectively.

In earlier diagnostic systems, such as DSM-IV, obsessive-compulsive disorder was categorized as an anxiety problem, but in the later version DSM 5 has a separate category, OCD. Regardless of this, OCD is most often associated with significant worry and anxiety.

Depression

Even if worry is also an important thought process in depressive syndromes, rumination is usually the central CAS process. Even in the additional problem areas later discussed in the following sections, the emphasis is often on rumination.

Sven has been depressed for a long time now. It's not the first episode. He is convinced that he cannot really stand the Scandinavian darkness during the winter months. It is in the autumn that the depressions come. His father was also depressed and for Sven it is obvious that he has inherited a significant part of his father's depressive disposition. Sven has tried different medications, but he is not sure if they have been of any help, and he also thinks that the side effects have been bothersome, especially the sexual ones. This time it has been worse than usual. His marriage is in crisis. Sven's wife says that she is no longer happy in the marriage due to Sven's depressions and she wants them to decide soon with whom the children will live in the future and who will stay in the shared house. Sven is low on energy, so much more tired than usual and can barely drag himself to work. Once he is at work, most things go at a snail's pace. It's hard to focus on the work at hand. He no longer eats lunch with his colleagues and thinks that most things feel uncomfortable and meaningless. In the moments at home when he does not rest and recover, he is irritable and stubborn. He often asks himself questions such as: "When did everything really start to go wrong? Will I ever be myself again?"

Metacognitive therapy and depression

There are good reasons to try to develop more effective treatments for depression. Psychological treatments such as CBT and interpersonal psychotherapy, as well as antidepressants have a documented effect. Unfortunately, however, there is still a large proportion of patients, up to 50 percent, who are not helped and a very high proportion who have relapsed into depression within a year of completing treatment. There is hope that MCT can provide a significantly improved understanding of the central inducing and maintenance processes in depression and offer opportunities to intervene more precisely against these. Treatment studies so far provide some support for such hope, and it has been possible to demonstrate both a higher proportion of patients who are helped by the treatment (see e.g. Callesen et al., 2020a; Hjemdal et al., 2019), and that the treatment can be conducted effectively with surprisingly few sessions – about 10 sessions in a study by Winter et al. (2020), and that the positive treatment effects seem to persist over a long period of time (Carter et al., 2022b; Dammen et al., 2016; Solem et al., 2019). In a comparative study between behavioral activation and MCT (Schaich et al., 2023), the results appeared to be similar between the two treatments. Nevertheless, there was a slightly higher proportion of clients who deteriorated after up to 12 months follow-up in the behavioral activation group compared to the MCT group. In the study by Schaich et al., the effect sizes were lower than usual for both MCT and behavioral activation, probably because the client group largely consisted of severely depressed patients with chronic depression and a lot of comorbidities. Another comparative pilot study also showed equally positive results for CBT and MCT (Jordan et al., 2014). In that study, however, the therapists lacked qualified training in MCT.

A meta-analysis by Cano-López et al. (2021), regarding the empirical evidence for the metacognitive model of rumination and depression, showed *good fit* with the model and this applied to samples with clinical and non-clinical groups. The metacognitive model of depression has also been shown to explain the symptoms of postpartum depression (Petrošanec et al., 2022) and predict rumination and depressive disorders in adolescents aged 16–20 (Pedersen et al., 2022). In a smaller case series study (n = 3), the treatment has also been tested for type 2 bipolar problems where two out of three patients were recovered at the end of treatment and where all three patients were recovered one year after treatment (Callesen et al., 2020b).

CAS in depression

In the case formulation and treatment of depression, the focus is on rumination as a significant CAS process. Rumination has been shown to be associated with the onset and perpetuation of depressive states such as major depressive disorder and depression in bipolar states (Batmaz et al., 2021; Kovács et al., 2020; Nolen-Hoeksema et al., 2008; Papageorgiou & Wells, 2004) and in depressive disorders in adolescents (Pedersen et al., 2022). The rumination is directed towards the fact that one is depressed, towards the symptoms of depression and towards the consequences of depressive symptoms. With the rumination, you seek answers to questions such as "Why do I feel so depressed? What does this say about me as a person? What can I do to put up with the difficult thoughts and feelings?" Self-accusations, a self-punishing inner dialogue – "You have to blame yourself; you don't deserve to feel better!" – can occur and can take on a similar form and function as other types of rumination. In addition, rumination related to the theme of suicide may occur (see Chapter 2 and the paragraph "Suicidal rumination").

Worry also appears as a depression-aggravating thought process. "What if this never ends? What if I can't find my way back to my normal self? Will I ever have something to look forward to again?" Concerns can also be directed towards pending activities. "How will I manage to take care of the children when they come home? Will I be able to cook dinner for them? How will I manage to spend time with the rest of the family during the holiday? What if I become a really bad role model for my children by being depressed?" Of course, the worry can also be related to psychotherapy: "What will I do if this treatment doesn't work either?" High levels of worry have been shown to predict risk of postpartum depression (Osborne et al., 2021).

Threat monitoring in depression often occurs as scanning for energy levels, motivation and emotions. In general, self-focused attention becomes a safety behavior in depression. "Now when I wake up, how do I feel today? Am I still tired? Do I feel any joy about seeing my friend later today? Do I feel any motivation?" Rumination, worry and threat monitoring of emotions and energy levels means that attention is internally focused, on negative themes in one's own person and on the symptoms. Thinking becomes repetitive, reasoning becomes circular and conclusions about one's own person and about future opportunities become negative. Hopelessness comes as a result.

Regarding CAS behaviors in depression, various forms of avoidance of social contact and of activities are common. One purpose of reduced activity and increased social withdrawal may be to create more time for rumination and self-analysis. Other goals, along with resting and trying to sleep a lot, can be to save or recharge energy. Additional reasons can be to try to get a break from the thought processes that are perceived as painful and uncontrollable, try to get a break from rumination by sleeping or even hoping to sleep away from the thoughts. In addition, the reasons for avoidance and for passivity may be due to beliefs that the negative thoughts must disappear before the usual activity of the day can start or before positive social meetings can take place. Alcohol and other substances are sometimes used to try to improve the mood, to numb oneself or to interrupt the negative thought activity. Some clients seem to actively try to deepen their depressive mood based on the idea that this can heal the depression.

Metacognition in depression

Depressed patients have been shown to hold positive and negative metacognitive beliefs about rumination (Papageorgiou & Wells, 2001b; Solem et al., 2016). Metacognitive beliefs have been shown to be stronger predictors of depression than, as predicted in CBT, dysfunctional attitudes. Further on, metacognitive beliefs seem to predict dysfunctional attitudes on the cognitive level beyond depressive symptoms (Strand et al., 2024). Among bipolar patients who have recovered from depression, persistent anxiety problems have been shown to be associated with maladaptive metacognitive beliefs (Reinholdt-Dunne et al., 2021) and longitudinally, baseline metacognitions have been found to predict depression among bipolar patients at three month follow-up (Palmer-Cooper et al., 2023). A common challenge for therapeutic work is that those who are depressed initially often show low metacognitive awareness. Unlike those who suffer a worry problem as in GAD and are usually highly aware of their own worry process, those who are depressed may initially deny or not recognize themselves in the fact that they are ruminating. Alternatively, the client may believe that the rumination is part of the depressive symptoms and a biologically controlled process. In depression treatment according to MCT, some of the goals are therefore to increase the client's awareness of their own rumination and the negative consequences thereof. This is done by exploring situations of depressive mood and, based on these, to identify trigger thoughts and the client's rumination response to these. Positive meta-beliefs are about rumination as a necessary strategy to understand the perceived problems and the cause of depression, to be able to get out of the state. Negative meta-beliefs are those about rumination and worry as uncontrollable processes, sometimes about the rumination as a biologically controlled process that is beyond volitional control. Negative meta-beliefs about rumination as a harmful process for the body and brain and about depressive trigger thoughts as important and harmful also occur. The depressed patient may have an approach to the negative thoughts and feelings such as "as long as they are there, nothing else can be done. First, I need to have a clean and clear mind and get rid of my negative thoughts before I can get started on the day's activities and commitments". A person who is depressed tends to experience it from object mode. You relate to negative thoughts about yourself and your pessimism as to facts rather than as to thoughts that you can either be very involved in or choose to do nothing with.

Stress and exhaustion

Siv is exhausted. She has been on sick leave for a long time, but is still very sensitive to stress, and feels fragile and volatile. She tries to catch up on sleep and is careful to follow her body's signals about current stress levels. She has difficulty remembering things, difficulty concentrating and feels that she gets tired at the slightest effort. What used to be everyday routine chores, she now experiences as overwhelming projects. For Siv, there is a before and an after the exhaustion. Previously, she was ambitious, high-achieving and had an active leisure life. She doesn't recognize herself anymore and is convinced that her body and brain have been damaged by stress. Of course, she hopes that it will not be permanent, but often feels discouraged about this. She remembers that time before exhaustion with several important deadlines at work, the office being understaffed and with a new boss who was not experienced and competent enough. At the same time, her beloved mother was seriously ill and Siv needed to care for her as well. She didn't get enough sleep and rest, nor time for herself. She remembers the days just before her sick leave as if her whole organism was sounding the alarm. That she had "gone into the wall", or perhaps rather rushed into it, was a fitting expression of her condition. She is now careful to live a healthy life, and she devotes herself to mindfulness and restorative "feel-good activities" but feels impatient that the road back will be a long one. Both her doctor and psychologist say that she needs to be patient, that she should be vigilant about her body's signals and not move too fast with herself.

The S-REF model predicts that CAS leads to persistent experiences of stress and fatigue. CAS is strategies for coping with stress, strategies which unfortunately lead to continued and even worsening stress. Worry and rumination are energy- and concentration-demanding thought processes where attention becomes threat-focused for prolonged and recurring moments. When asking people who experience problems with stress about what stresses and exhausts them the most – "Is it an abundance of activities, duties, commitments and stressful life events, or *thoughts* of all this?" – many, perhaps most, answer the latter. Most of the time, even those who have a very challenging external life situation can state that worry and rumination add rocks to the burden. The client can usually confirm how the stress increases with persistent thoughts about how to cope and manage to keep up. Often, the experience of stress is also intensified by believing that stress is dangerous. The message that stress is dangerous, something to be vigilant on and careful about, has often been spread by various stress coaches and by representatives of health care systems.

However, it seems that stress is a poorly defined concept (Juul, 2019; Koolhaas et al., 2011; Rück, 2020). Both researchers and laypersons sometimes describe stress as stressors in the environment, such as poor work environments, incompetent managers, unhappy marriages, sometimes as overt behaviors we engage in: "We rush around, hurry, multitask", refrain from eating healthily and exercise, etc. At other times stress is described as what happens in our bodies when the so-called fight-flight response or fight-flight-freeze response is activated in demanding real-life situations. A major American study (Keller et al., 2012) that followed up on mortality data between 1998 and 2006 found an increased mortality rate for people who had experienced a lot of stress. However, this only applied to people who had a perception of stress as something dangerous. Among people who did not believe stress to be dangerous and who still had high stress levels, there was no increased mortality, instead the opposite. Could it be that, in the worst case, a health care system that spreads the message that stress is something dangerous contributes to people becoming ill and dying prematurely?

A diagnosis of *utmattningssyndrom*, exhaustion syndrome, has frequently been used in Sweden, even if it is not an international diagnosis according to, for example, DSM 5. Internationally, work-related stress and exhaustion are often described by the term *burnout*. However, it does not seem obvious that the phenomenon of burnout, which has been used since the 1960s, differs in any decisive or meaningful way from the diagnosis of major depression, see for example Bianchi et al. (2013, 2015). The Swedish National Board of Health and Welfare (Socialstyrelsen, 2003) has developed diagnostic criteria that have been widely disseminated in Sweden, but not internationally. In these diagnostic criteria, exhaustion is described as follows (p. 9):

> An obvious lack of psychic energy dominates the picture, which is evident in the reduced drive and energy, reduced endurance or prolonged recovery time in connection with mental strain.

Furthermore, symptoms such as difficulty concentrating, significantly reduced ability to cope with demands, emotional liability or irritability, sleep disturbance, obvious physical weakness or fatigue, physical symptoms such as aches, chest pains, palpitations, gastrointestinal problems, dizziness or sensitivity to sound, are reported.

The symptom picture described with the Swedish diagnosis of exhaustion syndrome overlaps predominantly or almost entirely with the symptom criteria that occur in other internationally occurring diagnoses, such as generalized anxiety disorder and major depression. Especially if you keep in mind that comorbidity is more usual than unusual among people who seek help. The symptoms described in the Swedish diagnostic criteria also correspond to the predicted negative consequences of CAS according to the S-REF model. According to Rück (2020), for example, it would not be possible to include the Swedish diagnosis in internationally accepted diagnostic systems because the scientific support for the diagnosis of exhaustion syndrome is too weak.

CAS in stress and exhaustion

People who experience problems with stress and exhaustion often also confirm high levels of worry, rumination, threat monitoring, thought suppression, and various forms of avoidance. A person who is stressed may worry about whether they will be able to go back to work, whether they will ever be able to work again, whether they will be able to cope with their tasks and their role as a partner, spouse or parent. You can also worry about your symptoms, your stress levels and the risk of overloading. Type 2 worry, i.e. worry about worry, as in generalized anxiety disorder (GAD), may occur. Rumination about the symptoms, the reasons why you became tired, as well as self-accusation, occur. Often, in a similar way as in PTSD and depression, there are beliefs that the brain has been permanently or temporarily damaged. Threat monitoring will be directed at energy levels, negative emotions and symptoms of stress, exhaustion and fatigue.

Not infrequently, some who experience stress and exhaustion problems have also received advice from health care agencies to be vigilant for internal signals of stress, fatigue, overexertion and incipient exhaustion. As in depression, common CAS behaviors are low activity levels, excessive rest, and social withdrawal.

Metacognition in stress and exhaustion

As with depression, the client may initially show low metacognitive awareness. The patient may be used to object-level dialogues about stress. Many clients are accustomed to talking and thinking about how external events affect stress, not how worry and rumination perpetuate stress. Furthermore, the client may be used to focusing on the fact that it is the symptoms that constitute the problem, and initially have more difficulty seeing that it is CAS and metacognitive beliefs that produce and maintain the symptoms. Positive meta-beliefs are about CAS as strategies for recovery and healing. Positive beliefs can be about worry/rumination as helpful to understand previous stress experiences, to anticipate future stress occasions and strains, and to prevent burnout and further damage from stress. Negative beliefs about worry and rumination as both uncontrollable and dangerous thought processes naturally reinforce the experience of stress. Spada et al. (2008) found in a convenience sample of 420 participants that dysfunctional meta-cognitive beliefs were associated with perceived stress, anxiety and depressive symptoms. De Dominicis et al. (2021) tested MCT for work-related stress problems in a feasibility study with four patients. In the study, stress was conceptualized in a similar way to anxiety in MCT for GAD, that is, as an emotional consequence of worry and other CAS. Problems with perceived stress, blood pressure and general mental health problems decreased significantly in connection with treatment. CAS and metacognitive beliefs were also reduced and in line with predictions from the S-REF model.

Sleep problems

The S-REF model predicts that worry and rumination lead to persistent negative affect and difficulty relaxing. Insomnia is about difficulty falling asleep, awakenings during the night, as well as premature awakening in the morning. Sleep problems are very common and the prevalence of insomnia in Sweden has been estimated to be about 11 percent (SBU, 2010). In a systematic review Buysse (2013) reported the prevalence to approximately 10–20%. Sleep problems tend to be long-lasting. Insomnia is associated with increased sickness absence, increased care seeking and social disability. Sleep problems have also been shown to be associated with increased morbidity and mortality.

CAS in sleep problems

In addition to the fact that worry, and rumination generally cause difficulty relaxing, those who have sleep problems often also start to worry about their sleep problems: "What if I don't fall asleep tonight either? I need to be alert and sharp tomorrow, what if I get too little sleep? What if my sleep problems will make me exhausted/depressed/sick?" Even during the day, such worry can continue. For some clients with worry problems, it can be scary to go to bed in the evening when everything becomes quiet and still, and you become alone with your thoughts: "What if the difficult thoughts/memories come over me when I can no longer distract myself with an activity?" Thought suppression can occur where the person with insomnia tries to shut out trigger thoughts about insomnia or other triggers. Not uncommon behaviors in sleep problems are alcohol, legal or illegal substances, as well as irregular sleep habits.

In line with what the S-REF model predicts, worry, rumination and thought suppression have also been shown to be sleep-disturbing thought processes (Galbiati et al., 2018; Schmidt et al., 2011; Takano et al., 2012). Frøjd et al. (2022) found in a sample of more than a thousand patients with heart disease, that worry, and rumination predicted insomnia. Clancy et al. found in a meta-analysis (2020) that worry and rumination are associated with longer sleep onset latency, shorter sleep and poorer sleep quality.

Metacognition in sleep problems

The predictions according to the S-REF model are that positive and negative metacognitive beliefs are also present in sleep problems. Anyone who has trouble falling asleep easily realizes that worrying about sleep problems only makes it difficult but probably answers that the worry continues because it is perceived as difficult to control. Dysfunctional metacognitive beliefs have also been shown to be significant in sleep problems (Galbiati et al., 2021; Palagini et al., 2017; Sella et al., 2019). Treatment studies of metacognitive therapy for insomnia have not been found in this review.

Prolonged grief

Torsten and Ulla lost their teenage son to cancer ten years ago. Life has never fully returned after this. The real joy is gone forever. Living on has no real meaning for Torsten. He does what he is supposed to do, and he gets by. He does his job, exercises regularly and continues his assignments in several associations that he is a member of. In social situations, he often feels like fraud, he thinks he pretends to be easy-going and just fakes it when showing interest in other people. He often thinks that he should have been allowed to leave before his son. It is not right that a young person who still had all the possibilities of life ahead of him should have to die of a pointless disease. He sees it as his responsibility as a loving parent to both remember and check if the memories of his beloved son are still intact. On occasions when he found himself laughing, he often felt guilty and started to criticize himself for being superficial and having stopped cherishing the memory of his son. There are times when he becomes unsure if he can still evoke the inner image of his son's face.

Grief in connection with the loss of a loved one is a part of life and is not usually regarded as a psychological or psychiatric problem. It is natural that grief remains for a long time and that one can also be reminded of it on special occasions, such as on anniversaries of the death, birthdays or special occasions when one used to spend time with the person who is now absent. However, grief usually subsides, and life goes on. For example, you may find that there are times when you feel both happy and sad at the same time. In the case of prolonged grief, this process of fading and reorientation does not take place; see for example Killikelly and Maercker (2018). The grief continues and it is difficult to feel joy and interest, difficult to engage in social activities, work and daily chores. Life can feel meaningless, and you can stop taking care of yourself in terms of healthy eating habits, exercise and restraint with alcohol. The S-REF model predicts that complicated and prolonged grief is explained by CAS and maladaptive metacognition.

CAS in prolonged grief

Worry, rumination and various forms of avoidance perpetuate sadness, anxiety and a depressive mood (Eisma et al., 2017, 2020, 2022; Wenn et al., 2019a, 2019b). The rumination and worry in complicated grief revolve around different ways of trying to make sense of the death, trying to remember the deceased and understanding how to move on in life. Attempts to maintain contact with the deceased through various rituals and the use of symbolic objects prolong grief, as well as various forms of avoidance and emotion-controlling strategies and thought suppression. Occasionally discovering that you are not thinking about the missing person or that you feel joy can be perceived as disrespectful or unloving. Avoidance can take the form of not planning for the future, not taking care of oneself and limiting one's social interaction.

Metacognition in prolonged grief

Positive meta-beliefs are about worry and rumination as a way of understanding the death. There may be beliefs that worry and rumination will help the person find answers and find ways to deal with the loss. Furthermore, there may also be positive meta-beliefs about CAS as strategies for maintaining memories, love for the missing person, or showing respect for the deceased. Positive beliefs about the importance of trying to push away certain thoughts, memories, or feelings may also be present. Negative meta-beliefs about both triggers and emotions as threatening and about worry and rumination as harmful and uncontrollable processes occur. Wenn et al. (2019b) found large effect sizes for MCT as a treatment for prolonged grief in a pilot randomized and controlled trial.

Pain, somatic problems, problematic health-related habits and behaviors

A few studies have investigated the importance of worry, rumination and metacognitive beliefs in pain problems. In these, it was found, as predicted by S-REF, that catastrophizing of the pain experience and pain intensity increases in association with CAS, and that positive and negative meta-beliefs are associated with CAS (Schütze et al., 2020; Spada et al., 2016; Ziadni et al., 2018). Schütze et al. (2017) conducted semi-structured interviews with 15 patients with chronic back pain and found concomitant positive beliefs about rumination as a way to find coping strategies for the pain and negative meta-beliefs about pain rumination as an uncontrollable process. Among 446 individuals who declared having received a fibromyalgia diagnosis, Tenti et al. (2023) found that negative meta-beliefs about worry and beliefs about the need to control thoughts indirectly influenced the intensity of pain through two mediating pathways: State anger and anger rumination.

Somatic health problems

Psychological functioning is of great importance in serious medical conditions and affects patients' quality of life and continued course of illness/ prognosis. Anxiety and depression problems are very common in chronic diseases and conditions such as cardiovascular disease and cancer.

Unfortunately, Ulf has suffered different health problems over the past ten years. Most recently, he has undergone treatment for prostate cancer. He has been told that the treatment has been successful. Despite the positive news, he thinks that the outlook in terms of health has deteriorated further. He worries about relapses, about having to go through new difficult treatments, and about how his wife will cope if he doesn't survive. He doesn't really dare to relax and doesn't dare to look positively at the fact that he's still alive. In some strange way, it feels like he would challenge fate by embracing a more optimistic view of the future. At other times, he believes that his negative mood may increase the risk of relapse. He often thinks about what he could have done differently and whether he himself contributed to cancer by not maintaining a healthy enough lifestyle. Some days he can't get out of bed.

CAS and metacognition in somatic health problems

In MCT, in contrast to some CBT models, no distinction is made between worry for hypothetical problems or for current problems, i.e. between realistic and unrealistic worry. The advantages of not making this distinction become obvious when the worry concerns current and realistic problems such as serious somatic illness. Even those who have a clearly elevated risk in connection with a medical condition can express that it would be a relief to be able to reduce worry and rumination. Worry associated with medical conditions can concern things such as when a deterioration will occur or if a procedure will be painful. The rumination can revolve around the possible causes of your health problem, what you could have done to avoid it, and so on.

That repetitive negative thinking such as worry and rumination (Trick et al., 2016) and dysfunctional metacognitive beliefs have a significant negative impact on both patients with medically serious conditions and their relatives, was shown by Lenzo et al. (2020) in a systematic review. Repetitive negative thinking and dysfunctional metacognition has been found, among others, in conditions such as cardiovascular disease (Anderson et al., 2019), the heart-lung disease PAH (Caldarone et al., 2022), MS (Heffer-Rahn & Fisher, 2018), Parkinson's disease (Allot et al., 2005; Fernie et al., 2015), ALS (Dodd et al., 2021), tinnitus (Natalini et al., 2020), after a stroke (Pedersen et al., 2024), persistent post-concussion symptoms following mild traumatic brain injury (Rauwenhoff et al., 2024), emotional distress in burns, plastic and reconstructive surgery patients (Taylor-Bennett et al., 2024) and chronic fatigue syndrome (Jacobsen et al., 2016; Maher-Edwards et al., 2012). Worry and rumination can be associated with impaired sleep and thus negatively affect medical conditions (Frøjd et al., 2022). Regarding health-related behaviors in general, Clancy et al. (2016) found in a systematic review and meta-analysis that rumination was associated with health risk behaviors such as alcohol and substance consumption, unhealthy eating, and smoking.

Wells et al. (2022a) and Wells and Faija (2018) describe a large, controlled study in the UK, the Pathway study, in which MCT is tested to treat anxiety and depression in patients with heart disease. Other psychological treatments, such as CBT, have only shown limited effect in these conditions. In a qualitative study in connection with the Pathway study, McPhillips et al. (2019) interviewed 49 patients in post-cardiac rehabilitation, all of whom also had anxiety and depression problems. They conducted semi-structured interviews where each patient's anxiety and depression problems were conceptualized/analyzed according to both a CBT model and the MCT model. The authors' conclusions were that MCT proved to be a more parsimonious treatment model logically and theoretically and provided a better fit with the patients' emotional experiences. In MCT, no distinction is made between realistic worry and unrealistic worry, which means that even if the risk of relapses and deterioration in the medical condition would be very significant and real, the goal is still to reduce worry, rumination and other CAS. In 2021, Wells and others (2021) reported results from the Pathway study. There were 332 patients who participated in the study, where one half of the patients had been randomized to usual rehabilitation and the rest to usual rehabilitation + MCT group treatment during six sessions. Adjunctive treatment with MCT outperformed usual rehabilitation and significantly reduced anxiety and depressive disorders with moderate to high effect sizes. Repetitive negative thinking and dysfunctional metacognition were also significantly reduced with MCT.

MCT has also been effective in treatment for anxiety and depression in various pilot studies for people undergoing treatment for cancer (Fisher et al., 2015, 2017, 2019).

Substance use disorders

Åke drinks too much and he is aware of that. Alcohol has ruined a lot in his life – he has a broken marriage behind him and bad relationships with his two children, who are now almost adults. In addition, he has often received

complaints from customers and various managers over the years. His econ-
omy is in bad shape. His doctor at the health center tries to support him in
getting to grips with his drinking and informs him that drinking affects him
medically in several serious ways. Åke often feels bad when he compares
himself to other people. He is ashamed of who he is and feels guilty about
everything he has failed to do in life. He is pessimistic about his chances of
changing something substantially. At times when he doesn't drink, he is
troubled by strong self-doubt, anxiety and depression. When he looks back
at various mistakes in his life, he comes to the conviction that he is no
longer capable of reducing drinking and changing his life. When noticing
cravings for alcohol, he continues with desire thinking and imagining how
nice it would be allowing himself to have a few beers. "Might as well drink
again and try to silence the nagging thoughts about why I lack the character
to get sober!"

CAS and metacognition in substance use disorders

The S-REF model stipulates that overconsumption of alcohol and other sub-
stitutes constitutes CAS behaviors in response to trigger thoughts and cravings
and can function as strategies to reduce other CAS, such as rumination and
worry. There is a strong positive correlation between, for example, alcohol
abuse and repetitive negative thinking, i.e. rumination and worry (Devynck et
al., 2019). In addition, there are studies that show that rumination increases
cravings and predicts alcohol consumption (Caselli et al., 2010), and that high
levels of worry are associated with alcohol consumption in people with problematic drinking (Goldsmith et al., 2009).

Spada et al. (2013, 2015) describe how CAS and metacognition in addiction
can be described in three phases: Engagement before, during and after an
episode. They describe how engagement in cravings before can be described as
desire thinking, a corresponding repetitive thinking process to worry and
rumination. If worry often starts with "What if …?" and rumination with
"Why …?", desire thinking starts with "If only …" and is perseverative
thinking focused on attaining a craved target. During the addiction episode,
positive meta-beliefs are activated, such as "taking the substance will reduce
my worry/help me control my thoughts". Over time and with escalating
addiction, metacognitive beliefs such as "Thinking about the substance will
make me use it" or "Once I start, I can't stop" will also develop. An episode
of addiction is often followed by rumination and self-accusation. Thought
suppression is common. These strategies exacerbate a negative state of mind,
and thus increase the risk of new cravings and more desire thinking.

Desire thinking

Desire thinking is thus a response to trigger thoughts and cravings for the
preferred substance. Desire thinking has been found to increase confidence

in *permissive beliefs* like for example "I deserve it" or "I can stop whenever I want", in alcohol cravings (Caselli et al., 2021). Furthermore, in longitudinal studies, desire thinking has been found to predict cravings and binge drinking (Martino et al., 2017) and relapse after treatment (Martino et al., 2019). Desire thinking has been found to occur in nicotine addiction, problem gambling and alcohol problems (Caselli & Spada, 2010), and the thinking style has also been shown to predict cravings in various forms of substance abuse (Caselli et al., 2013).

Both positive and negative metacognitive beliefs seem to play a role in relation to desire thinking (Caselli and Spada, 2010). Dysfunctional metacognition has been found to predict smoking dependence beyond other significant predictors, including the number of daily cigarettes smoked, the urge to smoke, psychological distress and distress intolerance (Khosravani et al., 2024).

In a systematic case series study of MCT for alcohol use disorder, Caselli et al. (2018) found preliminary evidence of positive effects of the treatment. In a pilot study of group MCT for alcohol use disorder (n = 7), Kroener et al. (2024) found preliminary evidence for the efficacy, feasibility and acceptability for the treatment.

Anger management problems

"Sometimes I just can't control my temper and the person who then continues to mess with me must blame themselves", says Ylva. I don't take shit and I'm not going to let myself be taken advantage of again. I have a good intuition for things like moods and gut feeling and whether people are honest or dishonest in what they say and do. I usually perceive that instantly in a social situation. I often think about those who have treated me badly and I try to be vigilant of people with similar intentions or personality traits. People are often deceitful, they say a lot of cute and nice things, but they only wait for an opportunity when you're off guard and show a weakness. Those who try to appear friendly are often the most deceitful. At the same time, I often feel horrible afterwards for losing my temper.

CAS and metacognition in anger management problems

So-called *anger rumination*, rumination over themes related to anger, has been shown to increase and prolong anger (Caselli et al., 2017; Lievaart et al., 2017; Rusting & Nolen-Hoeksema, 1998). The rumination can revolve around perceived injustices, people and situations one remembers and associates with anger, or around plans to retaliate and take revenge. Anger suppression seems to lead to emotion regulation difficulties and increase tendencies towards aggressive impulsive behavior (Martino et al., 2018; Selby et al., 2008, 2016). Positive metacognitive beliefs can be about the maintenance of anger as a strategy to increase the experience of vitality, agency, status or health, for example: "Anger helps me feel alive, powerful and important. Refraining from living out your angry impulses is unhealthy. The rumination and anger will help me to get rectification and justice. Showing anger will make others treat me with respect". Negative meta-beliefs may be such as "I can't control my anger cognitions and my anger". A perception such as "when I get really angry, I can no longer control my behavior" is experienced from an object mode rather than from a metacognitive mode, e.g. "this is a thought I have about my capacity to deal with anger". That is, an important principle in the treatment of anger problems is to increase awareness of the relationship between trigger and response to anger and that DM or postponement can be applied to the trigger/impulse. Salguero et al. (2020) examined associations between anger suppression, anger, aggressive behavior, and metacognitive beliefs in a sample of 947 students. They found positive associations between anger suppression, anger and aggressive behavior, and between anger suppression and metacognitive beliefs about, for example, the importance of controlling thoughts and whether the rumination is uncontrollable. The authors concluded that their data confirms the S-REF model as useful for understanding aggressive behavior.

Negative self-view and self-esteem issues

Vanessa suffers self-esteem issues. "I usually have good self-confidence, she says, but I find it hard to be kind to myself. I don't feel that I'm good enough and that I deserve love and attention from others. Many times, I'm confused about my own needs and preferences in relation to what other people want from me. I try to find my true inner voice, but I still have a hard time finding it. I'm very sensitive to the needs and desires of others and I'm often afraid to disappoint them. Sometimes I wonder if I really know who I am. I seem to lack an emotional inner core. It all feels so disturbing and mazy when I think about it. I've read about self-compassion and have tried to practice it. I still try to figure it out, but I'm not sure if it has been of any help".

The S-REF model stipulates that CAS leads to problems with self-esteem and to a negative self-view. For example, experiences of worthlessness are one of the diagnostic criteria for major depression. In social anxiety, processing of "self as a social object" is something central, together with the worry that you as a person will be negatively judged by others. Similarly, persistent preoccupation with thoughts of appearance defects is found in eating disorders and in body dysmorphic disorder, BDD. In other conditions, such as PTSD, stress-related problems or borderline personality disorder, there are often experiences and beliefs that the self is somehow damaged. Various forms of worry problems are often associated with a self-view of being fragile as a person and lacking sufficient resources to deal with difficulties in life. In conditions where a lot of control rituals and so-called *gap-filling*/control of memory images occur, for example in OCD, the effect on self-view is often a weakened confidence in one's own cognitive capacity. As described in Chapter

2, psychological/psychiatric diagnoses in themselves can be perceived as having an explanatory value. The problems the client is struggling with can be attributed to the diagnosis, and the diagnosis can thus constitute the client's model of their own mind. "It's because of my ADHD that I can't continue with a boring, but important task", "It's because my brain has been damaged by exhaustion that I'm so easily stressed" and so on. In a course of treatment with metacognitive therapy, these types of beliefs could be explored and modified with reattribution techniques. That is, it is possible to explore and try out an alternative hypothesis, that it is rather the CAS and dysfunctional metacognition that creates and maintains the emotional and psychological problems that the client experiences.

CAS and metacognition associated with negative self-view and self-esteem issues

Problems with self-view and self-esteem are related to the fact that CAS is to be understood as ineffective coping strategies that work poorly. This effect is thus an experience of unsuccessful self-regulation. CAS implies that attention becomes self-focused towards a form of persistent troubleshooting and towards potential inner threats among thoughts, memories, emotions and body sensations. Typically, people with various worry and rumination problems doubt their own competence, ability to cope with challenges in life, their social skills, memory, their own judgment, their own theoretical knowledge and their five senses. Instead of seeing negative thoughts about one's own person as temporary and passing inner events, the negative thoughts are experienced in object mode, as facts that need to be dealt with. Worry, rumination and avoidance also make it more difficult to stay socially outgoing, active and interested, which in turn results in fewer experiences of positive social encounters and a deepened negative self-image. Self-critical rumination together with dysfunctional metacognition has been shown to be predictive of negative self-view (Fearn et al., 2022; Kolubinski et al., 2019). Hagen et al. (2020) found among 726 participants that negative self-esteem was predicted by rumination in response to anxiety symptoms and depressive symptoms. They found that rumination thus constituted a vulnerability factor for negative self-esteem and that rumination was activated by metacognitive beliefs.

There are some psychotherapy approaches in which special interventions are used, which aim, among other goals, to improve self-esteem. For example, interventions such as self-compassion (Gilbert, 2010) or schema work (see for example Young, 2006) with the processing of childhood memories to compensate for past or present emotional needs that have not previously been met. In MCT, there are no direct interventions for self-esteem or self-confidence issues. Although it is understandable that maltreatment during childhood and adolescence can contribute to psychological vulnerability, the S-REF model stipulates that CAS and metacognition explain why the problems continue and do not stop when maltreatment is over. Studies show that the association between having been abused in childhood and depressive problems in adulthood is mediated by the thought process rumination (Raes & Hermans, 2008), and that negative metacognitive beliefs mediate the relationship between early emotional abuse, depression and anxiety (Østefjells et al., 2017).

Problems with self-esteem and self-confidence are understood in MCT partly as consequences of CAS and partly as new trigger thoughts. A person who enters a social situation with the image of himself or herself as untalented or uninteresting can respond to such triggers by increasing their worry, starting to monitor their own emotions and social performance, and engaging in various avoidances, such as standing a bit away or avoiding eye contact. Another option, the one that would be introduced in MCT, is DM and attention shifting. Is it possible to practice DM on similar trigger thoughts, refrain from CAS and instead try to engage in social behaviors and use external attention in such a situation? Can you continue social interaction even if you also have thoughts of being uninteresting, untalented or boring?

Since negative self-view in MCT is conceptualized as cognitions about one's own person and as products of CAS, the question can also be asked: Is there any point in defining oneself as, for example, uninteresting? Can you choose how you want to define yourself/how you want to think about yourself? Can you choose not to engage in negative thoughts about yourself? If I already know that I am uninteresting, why process the thought any further? Do I need to take such a thought into account if I find that I have no use for it? Sometimes it can be observed that holding on to a negative self-view works as a coping strategy with the goal of, for example, reducing worry about future failures in career, social life or love relations.

Personality disorders

Personality disorders according to the DSM 5 and ICD 10 diagnostic systems refers to persistent patterns of experiences and behaviors that significantly deviate from what is generally expected in the person's sociocultural environment. The pattern is expressed in areas such as cognition (the way oneself perceives and interprets oneself, other people and events that have occurred), affectivity (the complexity, intensity, lability and reasonableness of the emotional response), interpersonal functioning and impulse control. The durable pattern should also be assessed as inflexible and prominent in many different situations and contexts, causing clinically significant suffering or impaired functioning socially, at work or in other important functional areas. Furthermore, the pattern should appear stable and long-lasting and be traceable back at least to adolescence or early adulthood. The diagnostic systems DSM 5 and ICD 10 state that the view of personality syndrome should be dimensional, i.e. the behaviors, cognitions and emotions described there do not in any way constitute different categories compared to normal functioning, but rather as dimensionally different.

CAS and metacognition in personality disorders

What is described in the diagnostic systems as personality disorders is, according to the S-REF model, to be understood as an expression and consequence of CAS and dysfunctional metacognition. Intensive and long-term CAS entails self-regulation difficulties and inflexibility in terms of cognition, attention, behavior and self-view. Spada et al. (2021) found elevated rumination and worry among people with personality disorders in a clinical sample of 558 people. Compared to people without personality disorders, those with personality disorders also showed a higher degree of positive and negative metacognitive beliefs.

In personality disorders such as borderline personality disorder, repetitive negative thinking (RNT) (rumination and worry) occurs to a very high degree, which causes self-regulation difficulties (Cavicchioli & Maffei, 2022; Martino et al., 2018; Richman Czégel et al., 2022; Selby et al., 2008, 2016). Difficulties with impulse control and emotional regulation can largely be explained by intense and prolonged RNT. In borderline/emotionally unstable personality disorder, worry, rumination and threat monitoring often revolve around triggers related to themes of abandonment or rejection. The most difficult moments are experienced in object mode and with fusion beliefs activated, that is, as if trigger thoughts about being left behind are the same as being abandoned/rejected. Often, trigger thoughts are not even experienced as thoughts, but rather as very negative, significant and difficult to regulate emotions. Common experiences of emptiness among these patients can be understood as negative effects of the CAS.

Threat monitoring is both internal and external. Internal monitoring will be on body sensations, emotions and cognitions around the theme of abandonment/rejection. External monitoring can be on various non-verbal signals of significant others, such as tone of voice, gestures, facial expressions, all of which could be signs that a significant other has the intention to withdraw or to be dishonest. Self-harming and self-sabotaging behaviors, which are very common in borderline personality disorder, often have the function of reducing rumination and worry and regulating negative affect. A negative self-view is usually present and, as already been discussed in this chapter and in chapters 1 and 2, this can be understood as consequences of CAS. Negative self-view, in turn, can also constitute trigger thoughts in new situations.

In addition, holding on to a negative self-view can be a coping strategy. An example of negative self-view as a coping strategy can be a person who consistently identifies himself as unattractive and hopeless to regulate worry and to prevent new interpersonal disappointments. It is important to remember that with the S-REF model it can be assumed that similar coping strategies often occur at the procedural/non-declarative level and rarely constitute declarative verbalized plans for behaviors and cognitions. This means that one of the goals of the therapy will be to increase metacognitive awareness and to switch the dialogue up from object mode to metacognitive mode. The problem, as the therapist conceptualizes it and wants to convey, is not a damaged self, but the engagement in thoughts of a damaged self.

Examples of positive meta-beliefs are that worry, rumination and threat monitoring will increase personal security, help anticipate separations, rejection and thus help to cope with disappointments and emotional vulnerability. Worry, rumination and threat monitoring are also perceived as uncontrollable processes and as harmful to the mind. For example, self-harming actions can be understood as attempts to distract oneself from rumination and worry and thereby to regulate repetitive negative thinking.

In a study of MCT with 12 patients with a borderline diagnosis, all with experiences of sexual or physical abuse while growing up, Nordahl and Wells (2019) found that MCT was perceived as a helpful and feasible treatment intervention. During the twelve months of MCT none of the patients discontinued treatment. After the treatment and at follow-up after one year and two years respectively, there had been major reductions in symptoms in terms of borderline-related symptoms such as self-harm, suicidal thinking, negative emotions, interpersonal problems and trauma symptoms.

In a study of social phobia/social anxiety (Nordahl et al., 2016) in which cognitive therapy reinforced with MCT was compared with pharmacological treatment and with a combination treatment of drugs and cognitive therapy, the authors found that cognitive therapy reinforced with MCT clearly outperformed both pharmacological treatment and the combination treatment drug + cognitive therapy. (In that study, it seemed that the addition of drugs to the psychological treatment resulted in a poorer treatment outcome.) In addition to the diagnosis of social phobia, about half of the patients in the study also met criteria for the diagnosis of avoidant personality disorder. The patients with personality disorder seemed to achieve an equally good effect from the treatment.

Psychosis

MCT has been tried in several case-series studies with patients with psychotic problems (see e.g. Hutton et al., 2014; Morrison et al., 2014; Parker et al., 2020). According to the S-REF model, it is not hallucinatory experiences or trigger thoughts per se that create stress and emotional problems in psychosis, but instead the CAS and dysfunctional metacognition. There are many examples of hallucinatory experiences that can occur as normal phenomena. Nor do delusions by themselves constitute problems or define psychosis. People may have all kinds of beliefs, many of which are neither scientifically based nor need to be embraced by most of the surrounding culture. Believing in, for example, creationism, astrology or being a climate crisis denier, does not in itself mean that criteria for a psychosis diagnosis are met. In the case of positive psychotic symptoms, it is not the hallucinatory experience or delusion that is conceptualized as a trigger thought; instead it is the thought about hallucination, the *appraisal* (Hutton et al.,

2014). The trigger thought associated with a voice hallucination could be, for example, "What if other people see me talking to my voices?" or "Why do I hear voices?", "What do they want from me?" Based on similar triggers, an individual case formulation can be generated from the AMC model, for example, or according to case formulation as in generalized anxiety disorder.

CAS and metacognition in psychosis

Worry and rumination also occur in psychosis as problematic thought processes. As with other problems, CAS is predicted to cause, among other problems, emotion regulation difficulties and negative self-view, and as with other problems, CAS is conceptualized as being controlled by dysfunctional metacognition, processes that should theoretically be possible to modify. Thought control strategies in the form of thought suppression have been shown to exacerbate experiences of hallucinations and delusions (Hartley et al., 2015). In a study by Hartley et al. (2014) (n = 27), worry and rumination have been shown to predict psychotic experiences in the form of hallucinations and delusions. People with persecutory ideas and paranoid delusions show significant problems with worry (see, e.g., Freeman & Garety, 2014; Morrison & Wells, 2007; Startup et al., 2016). In a randomized controlled trial, Freeman et al. (2015) showed that problems with paranoid delusions could be significantly reduced through a short intervention to reduce worry.

Austin et al. (2014) investigated the relationship between illness development and metacognitive beliefs among 367 patients with first-time onset of psychosis. Elevated levels of metacognitive beliefs correlated with more severe and chronic illness development.

Sellers et al. (2016) found among 159 people who either had been diagnosed with psychosis problems or assessed to be in a risk group for psychosis development, an increased prevalence of dysfunctional metacognitive beliefs. Another finding was that negative meta-beliefs predicted anxiety and depression better than the frequency of positive psychotic symptoms in the form of hallucinations and delusions.

Sellers et al. (2017) examined in a meta-analysis the prevalence of dysfunctional metacognitive beliefs in people with psychotic problems compared to people with other emotional problems and with a control group without psychiatric problems. The meta-analysis included 11 studies and a total of 558 people with psychotic problems, 212 people with other emotional problems and 776 people without psychiatric problems. They found an increased prevalence of negative metacognitive beliefs in both clinical groups compared to the non-clinical control group and that the people with psychotic problems showed a higher degree of positive metacognitive beliefs compared to both the group with other emotional problems and the non-clinical group. The authors interpret the results as meaning that an increased prevalence of dysfunctional metacognitive beliefs seems to be something general in psychological problems rather than linked to specific problems.

Østefjells et al. (2017) investigated associations between the prevalence of early childhood emotional abuse, depressive problems, anxiety, positive symptoms, and metacognitive beliefs among 261 clients with psychotic or bipolar diagnoses. They found that early emotional abuse was relevant to later psychiatric problems. In addition, they found that the associations between emotional abuse and anxiety and depression were mediated by negative metacognitive beliefs and that the associations between emotional abuse and positive symptoms were mediated by negative metacognitive beliefs.

Impaired social functioning and reduced social activity have been shown as risk factors among people who are at risk of developing psychosis. Among 109 people who were assessed to have an increased risk of developing psychosis, Bright et al. (2018) investigated whether metacognitive beliefs predict reduced social activity. The authors controlled for other factors such as gender, cognitive schemas, severity of positive symptoms, social anxiety, and depression, but found that negative metacognitive beliefs about worry as an uncontrollable and dangerous thought process, best predicted decreased social activity. In the discussion section of the article, the authors reflect on the connection between negative metacognition and reduced social activity:

> Why should someone with such metacognitions show reduced social functioning? It is likely that believing that one's thoughts are dangerous leads to avoidance of situations that may provoke negative thoughts in an attempt to keep oneself and others safe.
>
> (Bright et al., 2018, p. 525)

A brief summary

MCT and the S-REF model have been applied when reviewing each disorder and condition in this chapter and in the previous Chapter 5. To a varying extent, studies have been reported that provide evidence of the importance of CAS and dysfunctional metacognition in the reviewed disorder or condition. For several of the disorders such as GAD, depression, social phobia, PTSD and anxiety- and depression problems in rehabilitation after cardiovascular disease, there are large randomized and controlled treatment studies that support predictions from the model. In several treatment studies MCT has surpassed CBT or other active treatments. According to the theory, with reduced CAS and modified metacognition, a reduction in symptoms, distress and functional impairment will follow for all the disorders and conditions that have been reviewed in chapters 5 and 6. In the next chapter, the state of evidence for the theoretical model and for MCT as a treatment will be presented and discussed.

7 The state of evidence for MCT

Evidence for the theoretical model, the S-REF

As discussed in the previous chapters, the theoretical model (S-REF) has been formulated with the goal of developing a psychological treatment with a clear research-base in experimental studies from cognitive psychology. The idea behind this has been that a more robust research- and theory-based model is needed to make possible a much-needed development in the field of psychotherapy. Such a development is necessary given that the treatment results with treatments such as CBT or PDT are usually far from satisfactory for large patient groups with various anxiety (Carpenter et al., 2018) and depression conditions (Cuijpers et al., 2021). For several conditions, treatment outcomes do not appear to have improved over the past 40–50 years; see, for example, meta-analysis of Öst (2008), and may even have deteriorated (Johnsen & Friborg, 2015).

The S-REF model has been tested in many empirical studies over more than 25 years (see for example Wells, 2009, 2019). Before the S-REF was formulated, the scientific field of cognitive psychology hardly influenced the field of psychotherapy, except that different schema models and models for associative networks to a certain degree were influential in CBT. The authors Wells and Matthews argued that the schema models could not explain the processes that govern how attention is used in emotional problems and what determines whether a person continues or discontinues their involvement in, for example, a core belief. Wells and Matthews also incorporated knowledge from experimental research on the relationship between attention and emotion, which shows that attention is largely voluntarily controlled. The S-REF model is a so-called top-down model that shows how metacognitive processes regulate attention and thought processes, which in turn affects the regulation of emotions and self-view. In the book *Attention and Emotion* (Wells & Matthews, 1994) the authors review the research that support their formulation of the S-REF model.

Dysfunctional metacognition has been found to be a transdiagnostic process in a range of psychiatric disorders, and as associated with the negative thinking styles captured by the concept of CAS (Sun et al., 2017). There is

DOI: 10.4324/9781003597100-8

also evidence of robust cross-sectional relationships between metacognition and both anxiety and depression in childhood and adolescence (Thingbak et al., 2024). Nordahl et al. (2023) showed in a prospective study that dysfunctional metacognitive beliefs predicted metacognitive strategies, i.e. CAS, which further predicted anxiety symptoms. Metacognition has, as the S-REF model predicts, been found in several studies to predict psychological vulnerability and symptoms better than cognitive content (Bailey & Wells, 2016; Bennett & Wells, 2010; Gwilliam et al., 2004; Myers & Wells, 2005; Myers et al., 2009; Nordahl & Wells, 2017; Spada et al., 2007; Strand et al., 2024). Dysfunctional metacognition has been shown to be associated with rumination and depressive symptoms in adults (see, for example, meta-analysis by Cano-López et al., 2021) and has been shown to predict rumination and depressive symptoms in adolescents aged 16–20 years (Pedersen et al., 2022) and to predict psychological distress among adolescents aged 12–13 years (Schultz et al., 2023). Targeting negative metacognitive beliefs in the treatment of GAD has been shown to reduce repetitive negative thinking and emotional distress (McEvoy et al., 2015).

Huntley et al. (2022) found among college students (n = 675) that metacognitive beliefs explained exam anxiety better than intolerance of uncertainty. Negative meta-beliefs have been shown to be more associated with the symptoms of GAD than, for example, intolerance to uncertainty (Penney et al., 2020). Negative metacognitive beliefs have been shown in a couple of studies to mediate the effects of cognitive concepts such as intolerance of uncertainty and clinical symptoms (Chen, Tan et al., 2021; Thielsch et al., 2015), inflated responsibility and clinical symptoms (Sassaroli et al., 2015) and perfectionism and clinical symptoms (Kannis-Dymand et al., 2020). Self-critical rumination together with associated metacognition has been shown to mediate the association between perfectionism and negative self-view (Fearn et al., 2022).

Negative meta-beliefs have also been shown to predict anxiety and paranoid disorders over time (Sun et al., 2019). Metacognitive beliefs that have changed during treatment seem to predict positive treatment outcomes better than altered cognitions (Nordahl et al., 2017; Solem et al., 2009). Negative metacognitive beliefs, worry and rumination have been demonstrated as central mediators also in transdiagnostic CBT (Muñoz-Navarro et al., 2022).

There also seems to be a direct relationship between metacognition and quality of life, where dysfunctional metacognition and corresponding CAS strategies have been found to be associated with lower quality of life and where CAS strategies mediate the association between metacognitive beliefs and perceived quality of life (Havnen et al., 2024). Dysfunctional metacognitions seem to be associated with emotional dysregulation among both clinical and nonclinical populations (Mansueto et al., 2024).

Regarding the negative effects of CAS, there is extensive research support for the negative effects of worry (see e.g. Davey & Wells, 2006) and rumination (Papageorgiou & Wells, 2004) on stress experience, emotional recovery and psychological vulnerability. Rumination as an emotion-regulating and problematic strategy has been associated with conditions such as major depression and depression in bipolar states (Batmaz et al., 2021; Kovács et al., 2020), depressive disorders in adolescents (Pedersen et al., 2022), anxiety, substance abuse, binge eating, and self-harm (Coleman et al., 2022; McLaughlin et al., 2014) as well as borderline personality disorder (Cavicchioli & Maffei, 2022; Richman Czégel et al., 2022). Desire thinking, another form of perseverative thinking, see for example Caselli and Spada (2015), has been found to increase confidence in *permissive beliefs* in alcohol cravings (Caselli et al., 2021). Furthermore, in longitudinal studies, desire thinking has been found to predict cravings and binge drinking (Martino et al., 2017) and relapse after treatment (Martino et al., 2019).

In addition, there is solid research support for threat monitoring/attention bias as a transdiagnostic factor in a range of emotional and psychiatric problems (Bar-Haim et al., 2007; Cisler & Koster, 2010; Staugaard, 2010; Techmann et al., 2010).

Evidence for MCT as a psychological treatment

MCT is currently an evidence-based treatment for several anxiety disorders such as generalized anxiety disorder (GAD) (Af Winklerfelt Hammarberg et al., 2023; Nordahl, Borkovec et al., 2018; van der Heiden et al., 2012; Wells et al., 2010), social phobia (Nordahl et al., 2016), post-traumatic stress disorder (PTSD) (Brown et al., 2022; Jericho et al., 2022; Nordahl, 2016; Nordahl et al., 2024; Wells et al., 2015) and depression (Callesen et al., 2020a; Hagen et al., 2017; Schaich et al., 2023). For meta-analyses, see Andersson et al. (2024) and Normann and Morina (2018). Interesting studies, several of which are comparative, also indicate that MCT seems to be an effective treatment for OCD (Carter et al., 2022a; Exner et al., 2024; Glombiewski et al., 2021; Melchior et al., 2023; Papageorgiou et al., 2018; van der Heiden et al., 2016). In two different randomized, controlled trials, Exner et al. (2024) and Melchior et al. (2023) compared MCT with exposure and response prevention (ERP) in OCD and both found that the two treatments were equally effective. In the study by Melchior et al., however, the therapists, who were trained in CBT, had an average of thirteen years of clinical experience with ERP in OCD, but no reported formal training or previous clinical experience with MCT! A similar situation with uneven competence among therapists seems to be the case also in the study by Exner et al. The therapists in that study were trained in CBT but lacked formal training in MCT.

Treatment studies for personality disorders, or in samples where patients with personality disorders together with other clinical groups have been included, have also been conducted (Nordahl et al., 2016; Nordahl & Wells, 2019). A large RCT was recently published (Wells et al., 2021) in which the addition of MCT to other cardiovascular rehabilitation surpassed traditional rehabilitation regarding anxiety problems and depressive problems in cardiovascular disease. Several treatment studies indicate that MCT may be significantly more effective than other treatments. Large groups of patients with problems with anxiety and depression could therefore be offered more effective treatment than with, for example, CBT, PDT, or drugs; see for example meta-analysis by Normann and Morina (2018).

Several studies indicate that the treatment effects are long-lasting at two-year follow-ups (Carter et al., 2022b), three-year follow-ups (van der Heiden & Melchior, 2014) and after nine years (Solem et al., 2021).

Although MCT has shown efficacy in these and several other conditions in repeated studies, from a transdiagnostic perspective it is misleading to limit the discussion on evidence to specific DSM or ICD diagnoses. Johnson et al. (2017) compared MCT as a transdiagnostic treatment with disorder-specific CBT in various anxiety disorders in a randomized, controlled trial. The results between transdiagnostic MCT and disorder-specific CBT were largely similar, but MCT had a better effect on personality problems and showed a faster effect on anxiety problems. The authors highlight the advantage of a transdiagnostic protocol that the therapist needs to learn compared to several disorder-specific ones. Metacognitive therapy is primarily an evidence-based treatment to intervene on the underlying mechanistic transdiagnostic processes beyond the diagnoses described in, for example, DSM 5 and ICD 10. It is a treatment that aims to radically reduce worry, rumination and other CAS as well as the metacognitive beliefs that have previously controlled the CAS. It is a model – the only one that exists and thus completely unique as a psychotherapy approach – designed to systematically target and modify dysfunctional metacognition. By reducing CAS and modifying metacognition, it is predicted that the symptoms will decrease, as well as psychological distress and functional impairment, and a natural recovery process will occur.

There is thus evidence for MCT as an effective treatment for large groups of patients with different anxiety diagnoses and with depression problems. In these and other studies, it has been shown that worry, rumination, other CAS and dysfunctional metacognition have been reduced. Thus, there are good reasons to assume that MCT should also be an effective treatment for additional patient groups where problems with CAS and dysfunctional metacognition are present.

8 Some common considerations and doubts about limited applicability

Is MCT too cognitively demanding for many clients?

William, in the example below, can be said to suffer from an anxiety problem that, according to MCT, is caused by excessive worry, other CAS, and dysfunctional metacognition.

William, eleven years old, is objectively speaking in a safe situation. Mom, dad and big sister are kind and caring. He seems to have everything he needs. He really likes his class teacher and most of his classmates. Still, he rarely feels safe and secure. He is afraid of the dark, afraid of dogs, afraid that there will be a burglary at home and that there will be a war. Above all, he is afraid that something bad will happen to his mother and father. He doesn't dare to be at home by himself, not even for short moments. His parents must often reassure him that they feel healthy and that they are careful when driving. William still sleeps in his mother and father's bed. He has been invited to friends' homes to spend the night, but usually declines. A few months ago, after a persuasion campaign by his parents, he agreed to try, but Mom had to come and pick him up late at night. He had not been able to fall asleep and thought that it felt generally uncomfortable and strange at his friend's house the later the evening wore on. Lately, he has shown more and more reluctance to go to school. Mum and Dad have often pondered the background to William's fears. Did the adaptation to preschool go too fast? Is it related to the fact that William's grandmother died of cancer four years ago? A cousin of his grandmother is said to have been schizophrenic. Is there a genetic influence from there? Could William perhaps suffer from any neuropsychiatric problems?

From what ages can people usually understand the principles of metacognitive therapy? Köcher et al. (2021) found in a systematic literature review and meta-analysis that metacognitive beliefs in children and adolescents can be measured from the age of seven and up, and that these beliefs co-vary with anxiety and worry. One conclusion they came to was that the metacognitive model seems to be applicable to generalized anxiety disorder in children and adolescents. Esbjørn et al. (2015) found that the metacognitive model with some adaptations can be used for children with anxiety

DOI: 10.4324/9781003597100-9

problems from about seven years of age. Esbjørn et al. (2018) tried MCT for children with generalized anxiety disorder, 7–13 years old, and found that the treatment was feasible and seemed promising. In the book (in Danish) *Metacognitive Therapy for Children with Anxiety* (Esbjørn et al., 2016), they describe the treatment procedures in detail.

The S-REF model predicts that cognitive abilities will be strained during CAS. This is reflected in clinical situations where, for example, people with intense and prolonged worry may describe difficulties in concentrating and focusing on intellectually demanding tasks. It is not entirely unusual for clients with worry problems to also have suspected that they may suffer ADHD, but then, after successful MCT, to discover that the previous problems of concentration have disappeared together with the worry. Correspondingly, cognitive abilities are impaired during prolonged and intensive rumination. CAS is cognitively resource-demanding and thus exhausting. In addition, worry and rumination are thought processes that are biased towards the negative and threatening. Through the interventions in MCT, which, among other goals, aim to reduce CAS, the individual gains increased access to his or her cognitive capacity. Considering studies that have been published so far, it is evident that metacognitive dialogues and interventions work also in conditions when cognitive abilities are strained or where the cognitive level has not yet fully matured developmentally. It is important to keep in mind that MCT is not primarily about talking about or thinking about problematic thinking but is very much based on experiential exercises where the client is given the opportunity to experience and discover that the thinking can be regulated. In MCT, it is assumed that the individual already has an ability to reduce CAS. The experiments in MCT are designed to create opportunities to rediscover those abilities. Interventions that help the individual to interrupt worry and rumination early in the treatment lead to a release of cognitive capacity and a shift in attention and thinking to other areas in life than mental threat scenarios. As already mentioned in Chapter 6, metacognitive therapy has also been tested in pilot studies with psychosis problems (Hutton et al., 2014; Morrison et al., 2014) and for people assessed as having a very high risk of psychosis (Parker et al., 2020). In these studies, MCT has been found to be a feasible, meaningful and promising treatment.

Too simplifying? Is MCT a shallow kind of treatment?

Practicing *detached mindfulness* (DM) and postponing worry, could at first be perceived as an avoidant approach. The immediate associations can go to such as turning a blind eye to real problems that need to be dealt with. Several psychotherapy models, both in CBT and PDT, rest on the idea that losses, disappointments and traumatic experiences need to be processed. Many of the traditional psychotherapy models have encouraged increased introspection regarding traumatic memories, negative emotions, physiology, motivation, energy levels, thoughts or the "true self". In other evidence-based treatments for PTSD, it has even been seen as necessary to process trauma memories, which is something that does not occur as a treatment element in MCT. Initially, MCT may thus appear as an almost "anti-psychotherapeutic" model with the message "let your thoughts and emotions regulate themselves".

However, the experience of clients and clinicians is not usually that the treatment is superficial, shallow or reductionistic. Instead, MCT tends to be perceived as a fascinating model that provides the opportunity for new discoveries about how one's own mind works and can be regulated. The model does not only mean that the client discovers that worry-related thoughts about, for example, possible illness can be left alone for a while. In a similar way, examples such as negative self-view are also thoughts that can be related to in different ways. MCT also encourages some introspection in the sense that it is important to increase the patient's metacognitive awareness. In the therapeutic dialogue and through various experiments, the triggers that occur in a problematic situation and how the client responds to the triggers are explored. In addition, the emotional consequences of CAS are examined, and the client's metacognitive beliefs are explored and challenged. This type of introspection is not about continuously, for long periods of time, scanning or "processing" emotions, thoughts, motivations or memories. MCT is not about increasing self-focused attention.

Dealing with problems without worry and rumination

If MCT were to be perceived as a form of psychotherapy that propagates avoidance or problem denial, it is important to return to the question of mode, i.e. is the dialogue at that time in object mode or metacognitive mode? In MCT, we examine how the individual relates to thoughts about different problems, and usually you discover that overthinking in the form of worry and rumination is something completely different from effectively dealing with real problems. Paradoxically, worry and rumination usually lead to passivity and feelings of powerlessness, rather than problem-solving. The effects of worry and rumination are often that the individual feels more entangled in their problems, paralyzed, insecure, weak and dejected. Worry is often about thinking of problems that do not yet exist in the world. Rather, a more effective way to tackle really challenging problems is to take breaks from your thoughts. Sometimes the problems disappear on their own. Sometimes they are perceived as far less difficult after a break from thoughts. A person who has doubted his or her own ability to deal with a problem, when the dialogue has been switched up to metacognitive mode, can more easily discover that self-doubt is just more thoughts. After a rest from the thoughts, it is easier to gain new perspectives and ideas and to tackle the problems that need to be dealt with more effectively.

You don't become insightful, revitalized or creative by engaging in worry or rumination. Thinking is an instrument that is useful in some situations and problematic in others. People with mental illness can sometimes experience it as a very complicated project to get out of bed in the morning, take a walk and buy some food at the nearest grocery store, or to get around by public transport. The idea of bumping into an acquaintance during the walk or in the store can be perceived as a complicated scenario that requires a lot of preparation and planning. In object mode, everyday events and trivial tasks can be perceived as complex, demanding and burdensome. When shifting to a metacognitive dialogue, it is easier to realize that it is the negative and repetitive thinking that complicates life and that the only real problem is overthinking.

Transition processes after difficult events

In MCT, the starting point is that adjustment processes after difficult events in life are best regulated without attempts to control thoughts and feelings. Many of the symptoms after psychological trauma, such as intrusive memories and nightmares, can be understood as part of a completely normal, healthy and automatic adjustment process, *the reflexive adaptation process* (RAP) (Wells, 2009). According to the S-REF model, PTSD for example, develops in cases where this natural healing/adjustment process is disrupted by CAS. In a similar way, you can look at reactions after other difficult events in life, such as grief after severe losses. Grief is to be understood as a very natural experience and part of a process of adjustment. If grief is managed with CAS, the risk of it turning into what is known as "prolonged grief" increases.

Pessimism and hopelessness

Anyone who has had a lot of setbacks and who has become pessimistic can be helped to see that pessimism and hopelessness are perpetuated by rumination and worry. Behind a pessimistic attitude to life there may also be positive meta-beliefs about pessimism as helpful or protective. Through DM and by taking breaks from pessimism, life seems less dark and new opportunities become easier to discover. Anyone who persistently ponders the meaning of life and whether it is worth living on, can be helped to see that these are issues that can be dealt with at the object level or at the metacognitive level. Persistently continuing with the questions at the object level leads to paradoxical effects, that is, life feels even more meaningless, lonely, confusing and insecure. Dealing with the questions on a metacognitive level enables other conclusions, such as "These thoughts don't lead me forward. It is rather the thought activity that is meaningless, not life itself".

Stress

Stress is a normal and functional reaction to various strains in life. The stress reaction sharpens the senses and gives us the strength to do what we need to do in real-life situations. Stress and fatigue are normally transient in a similar way to other internal events. According to MCT, stress or exhaustion is not explained by being active during the day, having work-intensive periods in life, standing up for our fellow human beings or taking on new and demanding challenges. In general, such things tend to be healthy, stimulating and an aid to personal development. Nor is exhaustion explained by the fact that we have failed to monitor our energy levels to a sufficient extent or analyze whether what we do feels pleasurable or not. Negative life events such as divorce, death in the family circle or serious illnesses of our loved ones require our attention, time and energy, but do not normally make us chronically exhausted. Those who nevertheless tire themselves out by avoiding taking care of their own basic needs for sufficient sleep and rest, often do so out of concern that others, for example, might become dissatisfied. That is, even in such a case, it is worry that worsens the fatigue and impedes normal self-regulation and recovery.

The experience of stress is perpetuated and reinforced if we worry that our brains have been temporarily or permanently damaged by stress. Of course, it is a frightening thought if you believe in it and find it important. Worry, rumination and other CAS backfire and prolong the stress experience. Negative metacognitive beliefs, i.e. believing that worry and rumination are both uncontrollable and dangerous, result in increased and prolonged stress.

Loneliness

Involuntary loneliness has been identified as a risk factor for deteriorating health and increased mortality; see, for example, meta-analysis by Holt-Lunstad et al. (2015) and systematic review by Leigh Hunt et al. (2017). At the same time, loneliness is largely a psychological phenomenon. For example, many people may feel lonely in their marriage. Others may feel lonely and isolated at a party. When exploring loneliness as a psychological experience, the S-REF model would predict that worry and rumination lead to self-focused attention and reduced tendencies to social activity, and that these thought processes also will increase the experience of loneliness. If you instead interrupt self-focused attention, worry and rumination, social interaction will be facilitated. In the absence of repetitive negative thinking, it becomes easier to take social initiatives yourself as well as to respond to those that come from others.

Challenges in the family, in love relationships, at work, in society

MCT is not about turning a blind eye to problems that exist in family life, in relationships, in working life or in society. Denying the problems in our lives would rather be conceptualized as avoidance. Neither is MCT about trying to cheer yourself up when you are unhappy or about avoiding negative emotions. Reflecting on one's own life choices or how one feels about each other in a relationship is of course not in itself rumination or worry, although such activity could of course easily turn into worry and rumination. What is meant by CAS is precisely repetitive and persistent negative thinking.

In the following paragraphs, the discussion is further developed about MCT as anything but a superficial, shallow or reductionistic model. Instead, it is claimed that the model is profound and comprehensive in the sense that it has bearing on such things as creativity, vitality, focus and perseverance. The model is also relevant even for problems that at first glance do not seem to appear as thinking problems. "Not everything is thoughts, is it?" is one of the headings that follows. Furthermore, it is discussed how the model is relevant to problems that seem to originate from negative relationship experiences from early in life, for what are called attachment problems and personality-related problems.

On creativity, vitality, focus and perseverance

Clients often seek psychological treatment for problems such as anxiety, depression or negative self-image. Many also seek psychological counselling based on a feeling of not really using their own potential. It can be such as underperformance in studies and work, procrastination, restrained creativity, or not daring to accept opportunities in terms of love relationships, work or positions of trust. Behind inhibited creativity or the experience of not daring, CAS is most often found in the form of worry, rumination and various forms of avoidance. Again, given that worry and rumination are tiring and demanding processes and associated with psychological distress, it is understandable that creativity is negatively affected and that different projects feel less enjoyable. The person who starts dating can worry about all sorts of things about the new person and the relationship and thus find it difficult to stay open to the possibility, see how it all develops and take one step at a time. A persistent worry of failure makes it harder to stay positive, find confidence, see opportunities, and view natural setbacks as important and useful learning opportunities. Sometimes CAS occurs in the form of self-sabotaging behaviors, driven by the worry of failure or even by the worry of success. Inhibited creativity and underperformance can sometimes also be explained by behavior that has become emotionally influenced, i.e. behavior that is controlled by excessive monitoring of emotions and motivation. Most of the time, performance and perseverance are promoted by start and stop signals for the behavior related to the weekday and time of the day, rather than to emotions and motivation. CAS also means that attention is focused on potential threats instead of on the task to be performed, which will be perceived as disrupting focus, concentration and endurance.

A person who interrupts CAS will be able to allocate significantly more energy and attention to life's tasks, problems, challenges and opportunities. It becomes easier to realize that a thought like "I can never do this" can be dealt with as a trigger, that is, not at all (DM) or with postponement, for example "I'll find that out later when I have tried, for now I'll do the best I can". Greater opportunities are created to learn empirically from the natural feedback that results from trying new approaches. It becomes more natural to get involved in family life, in work tasks and in other social encounters. It will be easier to have a balanced and flexible focus, to pay attention to the opportunities and joys in life, not one-sidedly potential threats and dangers. To let your thoughts alone for a while is to give the brain much-needed rest and recovery. The chances of being able to sleep well increase. All of this creates increased space for more positive, engaged, and deepened inter-personal relationships. For example, Strand et al. (2018) and Strand and Nordahl (2024) showed that interpersonal relationships in depression and in other common mental disorders improved significantly after treatment with MCT. It is interesting in this context that the treatment did not include any targeted interventions to affect interpersonal functioning. A great many human activities work best with reduced thinking.

But aren't emotional problems more than thoughts?

Humans are complex beings and react with emotions, physiology and habi-tual patterns of behavior that they far from always reflect on or describe verbally to themselves or others. The view of problems that were initially experienced as "difficult emotions" rather than as thought problems was described in Chapter 2 under a special heading about emotions in metacog-nitive therapy. Based on the S-REF model, it can be discovered that emotions include a cognitive component, and that the client reacts with CAS to their emotions. Much happens unconsciously and wordlessly, at the procedural level. We have a history, both as a species and as individuals. Large parts of our brains are made up of evolutionarily older structures from a time before we evolved into thinking, reasoning, and verbally speaking beings. Largely, operations such as basic bodily functions are regulated from the brain without any direct involvement of thinking. Like other species, we have an inherited predisposition to detect and predict threats and danger and to react with a fight-flight-freeze response. Similarly, there are inherited predispositions for what we need to approach, such as community, sex, food, and many of these systems work without the involvement of verbalized thoughts.

As the herd-living species that humans are, there are also inherited pre-dispositions to social interaction, cooperation, social order and for forming emotional bonds. Being excluded from group membership means danger and stress for every herd-living mammal. Many of our individual patterns of behavior have been conditioned and shaped in early encounters with our closest caregivers, during periods of our lives when we had not yet con-quered verbal language and more sophisticated thinking. From the very first day of life, we try to influence our caregivers and allow ourselves to be influenced by them. A lot has been learned during a time in life when we were totally at the mercy of the caregivers' ability to give us security, guidance and good physical and emotional care for our survival. Essential parts of this early learning in life take place before the verbal language has developed. What we have learned in social interactions throughout life is largely wordless, so-called procedural knowledge. Attachment theory and theories about different attachment patterns elaborate on this.

Can MCT be helpful for those with negative relationship experiences from early on in life?

Attachment theory (see, for example, Bowlby, 1969) is based on observations that evolution has favored mammalian juveniles who sought the protection of their parents when required. Corresponding tendencies in parents, i.e. different forms of supervision, care and protective behavior, have also been favored during evolution. Attachment theories concerning humans describe attachment patterns both as external behaviors and internal psychological processes at the declarative and procedural levels. The attachment theories have developed both from animal studies and from studies of human children who have been separated from their parents for various reasons.

In the literature on attachment in the human child, it is often described how innate temperament differences in both children and parents interact with the quality of the relationship they develop. In addition, it describes how the attachment experiences that parents themselves have had, in turn, affect their ability to provide good care for their child. Secure and insecure relationship patterns early in life seem to constitute later models for relationship building. These experiences turn into positive and negative expectations for close relationships. Not having experienced a secure and loving emotional bond with the parents early in life leaves its mark and makes it more difficult to develop good and secure relationships later in life. Much of this is done wordlessly and is to be seen as procedural knowledge. The little abandoned child does not have the ability to reflect at a declarative level on "Mom and dad seem to have too big problems of their own to be able to take care of me in a good and affectionate way".

In a cross-sectional study in the general population (n = 304), Horváth et al. (2024) found a dose–response relationship between adverse childhood experiences and dysfunctional metacognition. Although many experiences of social interaction from early life can be understood as wordless procedural knowledge, the MCT model does not lack opportunities for intervention. As mentioned earlier, there are studies that show that the associations between abuse from early life and later psychological problems are mediated by rumination (Deguchi et al., 2021; Raes & Hermans, 2008) and dysfunctional metacognition (Mansueto, Caselli et al., 2019; Østefjells et al., 2017). A person who is aware of a lack of trust and negative expectations associated with social interaction can often describe stress and anxiety relating to interpersonal relationships. Often it is a fear of being abandoned, rejected, exploited or deceived. Seemingly impulsive behaviors often occur, where the fear of being abandoned or mistreated initially is not even conscious or verbalized. Not uncommon are behaviors such as breaking up a relationship prematurely, before nothing bad has happened or not attending meetings that would lead to opportunities for close relationships. Sometimes avoidance takes the form of not clearly expressing what you think and wish about another person, for fear of being mocked. Sometimes fear can manifest itself as a diffuse discomfort of getting too close to others, or as a sarcastic or prickly style of interaction. Anyone who in adulthood shows negative expectations in interpersonal relationships can be helped through an exploratory dialogue that is switched up from the object level to the metacognitive level. Whether the expectations are formulated in words and thoughts or manifested as more procedural knowledge, one could see all this as cognitions about bad things that can occur when relating to other people. Preconscious thoughts of painful events that can occur when socializing can be reformulated in terms of trigger thoughts and CAS in relation to the trigger. Trigger thoughts and worries can in such situations be about being abandoned, deceived or mistreated. The trigger and worry can also be related to the emotional reaction itself, such as "What if I get so sad that I never get over it?", "What if I will feel ashamed and feel stupid for having dared to hope?" or "What if I will be broken by negative emotions?"

Negative expectations and stress about meeting someone can be understood and explored as worry. In many cases, the worry behind ingrained avoidance strategies is implicit and may seem to be hidden but will be possible to express and make explicit in behavioral tests where the person is encouraged to approach rather than avoid. To begin with, the approach could be done as a thought experiment, for example, "Close your eyes and imagine that you are doing the opposite now and approaching the person instead of withdrawing". Possible trigger thoughts behind the impulse to withdraw could be: "What if she perceives me as weak? What if he's one of those who just wants to play with me? What if I become completely dependent on him and he then abandons me, and I never recover? If he gets to know me for who I am, he won't put up with me. If I express what I think, he will think I'm unintelligent. It's just as well to avoid going on that date. I won't be able to feel natural and relaxed anyway". The therapeutic dialogue after trigger thoughts and worries have been identified, can then transition to how similar situations would appear if the client applied DM to the triggers and instead increased such behaviors that usually are helpful when one wants to approach someone, get to know them or maintain and deepen the relationship.

Often worry and rumination come together. "She looked pretty cool last time; she's probably just waiting for a suitable opportunity to dump me. What's wrong with me? Why don't I have more intensive feelings towards this girl? Does that mean that we are not meant for each other? Why am I so turned off? I will never be able to function in a relationship. Worst of all, she talks a lot. It's like she's trying to inspect and get access into every little nook and cranny of my mind. Why is she so inquisitive and curious? Does she want to try to find the remote control and then be able to control me where she wants?"

In the next paragraph, the discussion is elaborated on how the S-REF model and the principles of MCT apply to all negative thoughts, including ingrained declarative and procedural thoughts we have about ourselves and the world around us.

Personality, cognition about who we are and about the world around us

Linn wonders why she so often feels exploited and not treated with due respect. I'm perceived as positive, caring and generous, but my self-esteem is totally crap. Men I've been with have in the beginning made me feel attractive and special, but over time they have shown less and less care, interest and respect for me as a person. Some of them have been controlling and jealous and gradually they have begun to say very offensive and derogatory things about me. One of them really scared me after a while. It's not only these men, but I can also feel exploited at work. I'm a person who has a very hard time saying no and I don't know why that's the case. But of course, that's pretty much how it was for me when growing up. I didn't feel safe and there was no one at home who showed any great interest in my needs, my thoughts and feelings or what I wished for. Often, I felt that I was uninteresting and in the way.

Hannes has read about HSP, highly sensitive person, and recognizes himself to the letter. He says it feels good to finally get a diagnosis. As far as he can remember, he has been perceived as nervous, especially susceptible to impressions, different moods, subtleties and pain. He has always been withdrawn and very aware of risks. He is convinced that he was born with a nervous system with lower thresholds for different impressions and stimuli. He has learned to manage his high sensitivity by being careful not to overexert himself and to give himself lots of time and space for recovery. He has also become careful to consider which social meetings and activities really feel meaningful, comfortable and not too demanding and to only say yes to these.

In the S-REF model, no distinction is made in principle between "peripheral" trigger thoughts and those that can be perceived as more central and profound and that revolve around one's own identity. A person experiencing problems with procrastination of important work might identify a trigger as "I have no desire to get started", while a person with a negative self-view could engage in the trigger thought "If other people discover who I really am, they will despise me". Those with problems such as body dysmorphic disorder easily get involved in thoughts such as "I look disgusting". Some triggers, as previously mentioned, do not necessarily have to be consciously verbalized initially, and part of the therapeutic process will then be to increase the metacognitive awareness, by identifying these, how the person relates to them and through metacognitive processes makes them important.

An alternative plan can be drawn up, such as: "If I were to decide not to engage in the thoughts of being socially inferior or defective in appearance, what could be an alternative focus of attention? How would I use my attention if I came to regard similar negative thoughts as lacking importance? What can be alternative behaviors and alternative attentional focus that can promote social contact?"

How should one understand the concept of self-view? Is self-view something else than thoughts? Procedurally or declaratively formulated thoughts about who and what we are, how we have become the way we are and what our possibilities look like? MCT provides opportunities for dialogues about how we relate to our thoughts about ourselves and to experiment with the self-view. "Can I choose how to define myself? Do I need to listen to the thoughts about who I am? If I perceive myself as uninteresting, what is the point of engaging in such a thought? What happens if I instead ignore the thought of being uninteresting and at the same time try to behave in a way that I know is helpful if the goal is to increase the opportunities for an interesting conversation? If I were to see myself as physically or psychologically repulsive, do I need to care about that thought? What happens if I stop worrying about being repulsive or otherwise defect? If I have the view of myself and my brain as damaged after a psychological trauma or by stress, or if I think my brain is dysfunctional because of my genetic heritage, are similar thoughts of any help? I don't know for sure what my brain really looks like inside my skull, but that I think about it and relate to the thought of it as if it were damaged, sometimes becomes obvious". How we relate to the negative thoughts about ourselves has consequences for other emotional, cognitive and social functioning.

The S-REF model describes how CAS and metacognition will affect the image and thoughts we have about ourselves. Remember: CAS is understood as coping strategies that work poorly and that have paradoxical effects on stress and negative emotions. Negative self-view and a negative view of the world around us become a consequence of CAS. Those who worry a lot often experience low self-esteem. The consequence of worry and ineffective strategies to reduce worry is that you feel weak, fragile, sensitive to stress and so on. A person who is bothered by obsessive thoughts often develops a similar negative view of himself. The client's self-descriptions are that they do not feel competent enough to deal with the challenges in life, that they do not dare to trust themselves as sufficiently educated, that they believe that their memory does not work as it should, that they doubt whether they have seen correctly, heard correctly and so on. A person who ruminates persistently and isolates himself socially often feels confirmed that something is wrong in his own brain, in his own mind, in his own personality. Anyone who ruminates about injustice easily becomes cynical, loses hope in their fellow human beings, and often discovers that they, in turn, and in the eyes of other people, do not appear very friendly or interested. How reduced self-confidence becomes a consequence of CAS has also been described in Chapter 2 under a special heading there.

According to MCT, as previously discussed, holding on to a negative self-view can also be a coping strategy. In some clinical situations, such processes can explain so-called "resistance" in therapy, or therapy-interfering behaviors. For example, holding on to the image of oneself as hopeless or unworthy of a good life can sometimes be controlled by positive beliefs that a negative self-view protects against painful disappointments. Some clients with long-term psychiatric problems may say "my symptoms and my identification with the psychiatric diagnosis give me a certain emotional security and an image of who I am, and therefore I am frightened by the thought of change or of getting rid of the symptoms". Another variation on the theme could be "defining myself as a hopeless case keeps me safe and means that I don't have to worry about difficult expectations from others". Or "identifying myself as dangerous and frightening, makes others listen to me and respect me".

"Neuroticism" and *trait anxiety* are transdiagnostic personality factors that have been shown to be associated with vulnerability to various anxiety and depression problems. Nordahl et al. (2019) found in a study that both positive and negative metacognitive beliefs seem to be underlying mechanisms for the vulnerability that has otherwise been attributed to the concepts of neuroticism and trait anxiety. The authors also note that with MCT there are opportunities to modify metacognitive beliefs and thus reduce psychological vulnerability.

Will successful treatment of generalized anxiety disorder also be personality changing? Kennair et al. (2021) showed in a study comparing MCT in GAD with CBT, that successful treatment also reduced vulnerability factors such as neuroticism and at the same time increased protective personality factors such as extraversion and openness. Similar personality factors seemed to change with MCT.

As previously mentioned in Chapter 6 of the book, MCT has been tested with promising results for patients with a borderline diagnosis and with experiences of sexual or physical abuse during childhood (Nordahl & Wells, 2019), in psychosis problems (Hutton et al., 2014; Morrison et al., 2014; Parker et al., 2020) and in cases of social phobia among people with avoidant personality disorder (Nordahl et al., 2016).

9 MCT as a new paradigm and looking ahead

The theoretical foundation of MCT in relation to other psychotherapy models

Not only MCT, but also several other psychotherapy models, emphasize the relationships between cognition, emotion and behavior in relation to psychological problems. Likewise, there exist other psychotherapy models as well where some focus will be on processes such as worry, rumination, threat monitoring and unhelpful behaviors. In the following paragraphs, we will discuss how MCT relates to cognitive behavioral therapy and furthermore to what has sometimes been called "third-wave CBT", such as *acceptance and commitment therapy* (ACT) and mindfulness-based CBT.

Is MCT *an additional form of CBT?*

Some therapeutic techniques used in CBT are also used in MCT, but then they are delivered with a different rationale, i.e. with the pronounced purpose of modifying metacognitive beliefs. For example, behavioral experiments are used in both CBT and MCT. Exposure can also occur in MCT, but then with a different rationale than in CBT, and in addition, the exposure is not repetitive and long-lasting as in CBT. In the introduction to Chapter 3, several therapeutic techniques from CBT that become theoretically and clinically incompatible with MCT were also described. For example, in MCT, techniques such as applied relaxation, skills training, exposure to traumatic memories, questioning the evidence of negative automatic thoughts, cognitive restructuring of core beliefs/schemas, acceptance techniques or compassion-focused techniques are not used.

Both in CBT and in MCT, the role of cognition is regarded as important. There are also models within CBT that focus on the processes that in MCT are referred to as the CAS. In MCT, however, the focus is on how cognition is used to regulate cognition, i.e. on the importance of metacognition as an explanation for CAS and hence for psychological problems. In MCT, the processes referred to as CAS are explained in terms of dysfunctional metacognition. The focus of the therapeutic process in MCT is thus on

DOI: 10.4324/9781003597100-10

metacognitive change. In CBT, the corresponding processes to CAS are explained by different schema models or by respondent and operant learning theory. The emphasis in CBT is not on targeting, systematically exploring, challenging and modifying metacognition.

In 1994, the S-REF was formulated as a new theoretical model for psychological treatment (Wells & Matthews, 1994). It was described how the model was generated from information process theory and experimental research on attention, cognition and emotion. One purpose of this theoretical foundation in experimental studies was to provide a better understanding of transdiagnostic processes that lead to emotional dysregulation and psychological problems. Through an improved and empirically based understanding of transdiagnostic mechanisms, it was assumed that the conditions for real and much-needed development in the field of psychotherapy would improve significantly. In early publications from the 1990s, several of the current MCT models for the treatment of generalized anxiety disorder (GAD) and obsessive-compulsive disorder (OCD) have been formulated (Wells, 1995, 1997).

In 1995, MCT for GAD was described as "A cognitive model of generalized anxiety disorder" and in 1997 the models for GAD and OCD were portrayed in a book titled *Cognitive Therapy of Anxiety Disorders: A Practice Manual and Conceptual Guide.*

At least since 2009, Wells and colleagues have consistently defined MCT as an independent and different form of therapy to CBT (Fisher & Wells, 2009; Wells, 2009). Today, MCT should definitely be defined as an independent form of psychotherapy and a treatment model with growing scientific support.

There are several reasons to define MCT as an independent model separate from CBT:

- CBT is an umbrella term that encompasses several theories and thus constitutes an eclectic tradition. The S-REF model on which MCT is based differs from the theoretical models in CBT, which are more numerous and often mutually contradictory, and which are based on different variants of schema models or behaviorist models of conditioning.
- MCT is a strictly theory- and principle-driven transdiagnostic treatment. Techniques from other psychotherapy traditions are not incorporated in an eclectic way. The therapeutic interventions follow logically, based on the S-REF model, and are precisely targeted and aimed at identifying and modifying CAS and dysfunctional metacognition.
- One of the starting points in MCT is that cognitive content lacks significance. Instead, negative thought processes controlled by metacognitive processes are in the focus for treatment. In the schema-based CBT models, cognitive content is regarded as important to change in treatment.
- Negative self-view is understood in MCT as a product of the CAS, as further cognitive content and without any explanatory value. In the

schema-based CBT models, negative self-view is considered to have explanatory value and constitute vulnerability to psychopathology, and thereby a goal there is to intervene against thought content/negative self-view.

- Certain constructs used in CBT, such as intolerance of uncertainty, inflated responsibility or perfectionism is not given any explanatory value according to the S-REF model, but is instead understood as additional thought content, by-products of the CAS and of dysfunctional metacognition.

- In MCT, there are certain verbal and behavioral techniques that also occur in CBT. The rationale for the interventions in MCT is, in contrast to various rationales in CBT, consistently to modify dysfunctional metacognition. Many of the most common techniques in CBT are not used in MCT and are seen as logically contradictory, not compatible with the S-REF model.

Is MCT a form of "third-wave CBT"?

Both in MCT and in what has been called "third wave CBT", such as ACT or mindfulness-based CBT, the focus is on negative thought processes instead of thought content. This is probably what sometimes makes the models perceived as close to each other. However, any resemblance between the models is superficial. Mindfulness interventions in CBT are largely sprung from a Buddhist, philosophical tradition and are not founded as mechanism explanations from psychological theory. MCT is a highly theory-driven model where it is emphasized that the therapist needs to be in constant contact with and intervene based on the theoretical model, S-REF. ACT is based on *relational frame theory* (RFT) (Hayes et al., 1999), a theory of language and cognition derived from behaviorism and without any real conceptual similarities to S-REF. The treatment principles, interventions and rationale for the interventions are different in several crucial ways.

As mentioned in previous chapters of the book, *detached mindfulness* (DM) is a different intervention and another and more precise concept than Buddhist-inspired mindfulness. For detached mindfulness (DM), there is no prescribed ritual such as, for example, meditating 45 minutes a day for eight weeks. DM refers only to the relationship to a thought, that is, to note it as separate from the self and for the moment to refrain from further involvement in it. DM is the antithesis of CAS. Body scanning, use of "breathing anchor", or instructions to be in contact with *the present moment* are procedures occurring in Buddhist-inspired mindfulness, but that are not used when introducing and practicing DM. Acceptance as a concept becomes theoretically superfluous in MCT and is not used as an intervention.

MCT as a new paradigm for psychological treatment

Can MCT more effectively explain the psychological problems and how they can be treated? There are several evidence-based psychological treatments for different types of problems and diagnoses. One thesis in MCT is that the mechanisms of action in all psychological treatment that works consist of CAS and dysfunctional metacognition in some way being changed and reduced. In psychotherapies with successful treatment outcomes, this is mostly assumed to have occurred indirectly, unintentionally and unsystematically. MCT has been developed to precisely and systematically identify and directly reduce the presumed causal mechanisms of mental illness, i.e. CAS and dysfunctional metacognition.

To summarize from previous chapters: The theoretical and clinical approach is that MCT can constitute a new paradigm for psychological treatment and through a stronger empirically based theory be able to stimulate research and much-needed development in the field of psychotherapy. Although there are currently effective psychological treatments for various disorders, the proportion of clients who are recovered or long-term helped is far from satisfactory (Baker et al., 2021; Carpenter et al., 2018; Cuijpers et al., 2021). There is a hope that treatment outcomes can be significantly improved with the help of a stronger theory. The S-REF model is designed to enable treatment of a wide range of psychological problems and provide improved precision in terms of analysis and interventions. The model is also developed to provide more precise understanding and effective interventions in comorbid problems. The predictions that can be made according to S-REF are researchable, possible to subject to empirical testing.

In chapters 5 and 6 we reviewed how MCT can increase the understanding and treatment options for a wide variety of common disorders and psychological problems. In Chapter 7, the state of evidence for the S-REF model and for MCT as a treatment was presented.

If further treatment studies confirm that MCT can outperform other evidence-based treatments, and if the theoretical model also continues to hold up to repeated empirical tests, MCT may emerge as an established paradigm for psychological treatment and treatment research. In Chapter 8, common initial concerns and doubts about possible limited applicability were addressed. In that chapter we also reviewed how MCT can also offer an improved understanding and targeted, effective interventions for many types of other problems, such as personality-related problems, relationship difficulties, involuntary loneliness, stress, underachievement, study problems, etcetera.

Regarding MCT as a paradigm shift in clinical psychology, Capobianco and Nordahl (2023) refer to "The Lancet Psychiatry Commission on psychological treatments research in tomorrow's science" (Holmes et al., 2018). There, Holmes and others highlight the importance of future psychotherapy research theorizing and clarifying the mechanisms through which therapeutic interventions operate. They advocate experimental research to identify these mechanisms. Capobianco and Nordahl argue that MCT as a model already exemplifies the desirable development in the field of psychotherapy that Holmes and others are calling for. They refer to the fact that a robust psychological theory of causal mechanisms was first developed experimentally then tested regarding the presumed mechanisms, and based on this, specific targeted treatment techniques have been developed and further tested empirically.

MCT *as a paradigm in everyday clinical practice*

As highlighted in several previous chapters, it is possible to see several advantages of transdiagnostic theory-driven treatment over diagnosis-specific therapies. With diagnosis-specific evidence-based treatments, it becomes very demanding for the clinician to achieve a high level of competence for the different treatments that can be applied to a wider range of common mental health problems. In addition to the fact that it will be difficult to develop a required high level of competence for many diagnosis-specific problems, it will also be demanding to be able to maintain and improve this competence in many treatment protocols. Another challenge with diagnosis-specific treatments is that the clients' problems are very often comorbid. Choosing which individual diagnosis to treat in that case will not be a particularly easy task for the psychologist or psychotherapist.

Not only for the field of psychotherapy in general, but also in everyday clinical practice, psychological treatment becomes problematic without a clear foundation in empirically based psychological theory. Treatment models that are characterized by eclecticism entail limitations. One risk is that the clinician uses different models for case formulations and interventions without being able to justify their choices based on a deeper theoretical understanding of the processes that are problematic and that need to be changed. Another risk is that it becomes more difficult to assess whether the therapist works sufficiently skillfully, consistently and systematically with certain interventions or whether, based on the clinical picture, it would be better to change track and try another intervention or treatment protocol. An eclectic model does not provide guidance on this type of clinical choice situation. Other risks are that the therapist only uses techniques that feel familiar instead of developing new skills and acquiring new knowledge that would be needed. In addition, there is a risk that the therapist applies interventions that are evidence-based for a particular disorder to a completely different problem where evidence for the intervention is lacking. If the psychotherapy model does not provide systematic guidance on how different clinical choice situations should be dealt with, the risk increases that the therapist will largely choose based on their own intuition and personal preferences.

Unlike technique- or module-based treatments from other psychotherapy approaches, MCT is, as emphasized repeatedly throughout the book, a theory-driven model. The treatment is not conducted according to modules for a certain number of sessions, but instead based on how CAS and meta-cognition change in the individual case. MCT prescribes how the treatment principles and interventions should be delivered and according to which sequence they should be implemented. The clinical choice situations for the therapist are fewer compared to other psychotherapy models. The therapeutic techniques used are fewer than in, for example, CBT. The theory is practically useful, distinct to the therapist who has been trained in MCT and necessary for the therapist at every stage of the treatment. The model is usually also perceived as very clear-cut and logical by the client. The MCT therapist is expected to be in contact with the S-REF model during almost every moment of therapy in an ongoing exploration of how the CAS and metacognition are expressed in the current case and in the current moment. The theory for the treatment in MCT is only one. The basis for the treatment does not lie in several and mutually contradictory schema theories and learning theories.

In clinical practice, MCT should have the capacity to represent a long-awaited new paradigm. Through the transdiagnostic perspective, CAS and metacognition will emerge in the foreground rather than specific diagnoses according to the DSM or ICD systems. For the individual psychologist/psychotherapist and for the clinic, it becomes a lot easier to stick to one model for treatment for most psychological problems, instead of having to educate oneself or the staff and maintain competence in many treatment protocols from different treatment models and theories. "Less is more". The psychologist Maja, from one of the vignettes in Chapter 1, and many of her colleagues will get new opportunities to deal with comorbidity and similar clinical choice situations described there. The psychotherapeutic techniques are relatively few in MCT and directly targeted – based on the current case formulation – at the causal processes beyond the DSM and ICD diagnoses. The model is perceived as stringent by most psychologists and psychotherapists that undergo training and supervision in MCT. The problems experienced by the client will appear as significantly fewer based on the S-REF model. They become clear-cut and easier to handle effectively when the therapeutic conversation is switched from the object level to the metacognitive level. It will be a lot easier to navigate.

Through the metacognitive dialogue and interventions from MCT, the client is offered opportunities to discover their own inherent ability to regulate emotions and thoughts. This discovery of the ability to self-regulate gives hope and increased confidence in one's own capacities. With this increased self-regulation, the problems and challenges in life become much easier to deal with.

Looking ahead

In an editorial on about thirty articles on the theme "Metacognitive Therapy: Science and practice of a paradigm", Wells et al. (2020) describe how development and renewal in the field of psychotherapy should benefit significantly more from a systematic theory-driven empiricism than through eclectic, technology-driven approaches. The authors describe that the development of MCT as a model has taken place precisely through the previous approach and not from integrative approaches with the incorporation of new techniques. The goal has been to develop a strong theory of causal mechanisms, grounded in cognitive psychology and cognitive science of emotion. Such an empirically based theory can provide better guidance in the exploration of transdiagnostic processes and the development of specific treatment techniques. The article in which Wells (2019) further develops and refines the S-REF model concludes with:

> Advances in psychotherapy require a paradigm shift; stronger information-processing theory that can successfully explain the control of cognition and the negative subjective changes in perceived control and sense of self that are central features of disorder. Psychological wellbeing is not a matter of what we think. It is an issue of how we regulate the cognitive processes that prioritize and extend thoughts. It is the stance taken in relation to the content of the limited capacity "thinking space". It is above all, the nature and effect of *metacognitive information* generated, held and used by processing systems.
>
> (Wells, 2019, p. 13)

Capobianco and Nordahl (2023) highlight the importance of theory and methodological integrity in further studies of MCT. They point to such as ensuring that future therapists have formal training in MCT and that competence and adherence to the method are carefully observed and followed up. They also point to the risks of dilution of the method, suboptimal treatment outcomes – and in the longer term misleading meta-analyses – if theoretical integrity is not maintained and if techniques from other psychotherapy models are used eclectically.

The current situation in Sweden is such that the Swedish National Board of Health and Welfare (Socialstyrelsen, 2021) generally recommends "CBT" as a psychological treatment for anxiety and depression states, without further specification about which treatment protocol is then referred to. Based on the discussion above about the importance of theoretical and methodological integrity and what has previously been stated about MCT in relation to other therapy models, it will be of paramount importance that future updated guidelines specify MCT as a distinct treatment method separate from CBT.

In a historical review of how MCT has developed as a psychotherapy model, Capobianco and Nordahl (2023, p. 16) write:

> After 36 years of theory and research, MCT is still in its developmental stages, and much remains to be explored, such as applications to occupational settings, physical illnesses, severe mental illnesses, addiction, and children and adolescents.

Capobianco and Nordahl, as well as Normann and Morina (2018) in a meta-analysis, note that although MCT in several comparative studies has outperformed CBT and control groups on the waiting list, there is a need for several larger randomized controlled studies where MCT is compared with other active treatment. Further major studies by independent research groups need to be conducted.

Meanwhile, awaiting additional larger studies, it can be concluded that MCT is already a documented effective treatment for very large patient groups. The model often provides completely new opportunities to understand psychological problems and to treat them. A shortcoming today is that too few clients have access to MCT because only a small number of clinicians have yet been trained in the treatment model. Many clients who have tried other evidence-based treatments without sufficient effect wish to try MCT. The need for education and training is great, and formal training is crucial for the clinician to be able to perform the treatment safely and with the intended high quality for the patient.

MCT as a treatment model is also interesting in that the model seems to attract both experienced psychologists/psychotherapists and relatively new graduates, and this also regardless of the therapist's previous theoretical background. The clinician's previous theoretical background does not seem to have any real significance, if there is a motivation to learn a new theoretical/clinical perspective. Many psychologists and psychotherapists with original training in both CBT and PDT have found that the model provides improved understanding, completely new tools in clinical situations and that it is applicable across a wider range of psychological problems. Hopefully, this book will be able to stimulate further interest, continued learning and more research and treatment studies.

Appendix 1: The concepts in MCT and their abbreviations

AMC model

is an analytical model in MCT where A stands for antecedent (the identified trigger thought), M for metacognitive beliefs and CAS, and C for emotional consequences or symptoms.

Attention training technique (ATT)

is a technique in MCT that is usually included in the treatment of depression. One purpose of ATT is for the client to have an increased experience of attention being under executive control, i.e. that attention can be flexibly moved from negative thoughts towards different external events.

Behavioral assessment test (BAT)

Behavior tests can be used where the client has difficulty describing symptoms, triggers, CAS, and metacognitive beliefs due to prolonged and extensive avoidance strategies. The client is then encouraged to approach the situation, which is usually avoided, to increase metacognitive awareness and to facilitate continued case formulation.

Cognitive attentional syndrome (CAS)

A characteristic of CAS is that attention becomes biased and persistently threat focused. CAS consists of repetitive negative thought processes such as worry and rumination, as well as threat monitoring and unhelpful behaviors and thought control strategies. CAS is to be understood as voluntarily controlled coping strategies.

Detached mindfulness (DM)

is the act of noting a thought, but for the moment refraining from further response or engagement in it. Detached mindfulness can be understood as the antithesis of CAS. In detached mindfulness the thoughts are experienced as separate from the observing self.

Exposure and response commission (ERC)	A form of exposure where a client with OCD problems is encouraged to keep the obsessive thought in their consciousness while performing the compulsive ritual.
Exposure and response prevention (ERP)	Exposure and response prevention or exposure with ritual prevention is a traditional CBT intervention or treatment strategy for OCD. In CBT, ERP typically involves intense, recurrent, and relatively prolonged exposure to anxious stimuli or thoughts while preventing compulsive rituals. The purpose there is for habituation to occur, i.e. for the anxiety to gradually decrease, or inhibitory learning, i.e. for the client to discover that nothing dangerous occurs when they refrain from rituals. In MCT, ERP is carried out in a significantly shorter time and less often. In MCT, the rationale for ERP is to modify dysfunctional metacognition.
Fusion beliefs	are metacognitive beliefs that certain thoughts are particularly important in the sense that the thoughts could influence external events. See below on thought action fusion (TAF), thought event fusion (TEF) and thought object fusion (TOF).
GAD	Generalized anxiety disorder.
Gap-filling	is a form of rumination that occurs especially in PTSD. Gap-filling means that the individual returns to memories of a course of events and tries to fill the gaps in the memories. Gap-filling is often controlled by metacognitive beliefs that more complete memory images would increase knowledge about guilt issues or that dangers can be more easily avoided in the future.
MCS	the Metacognitive control system.
MCT	Metacognitive therapy.
Metacognition	Cognition applied to cognition, thoughts about the thoughts or about the thought processes. Metacognition is the part of our thinking that regulates, directs and monitors cognitive activity.
Metacognitive beliefs	are different beliefs that the individual has about their thought processes and thoughts. MCT focuses on positive metacognitive beliefs about worry and rumination, such as "By worrying, I reduce the risk of accidents", and negative metacognitive beliefs about worry or rumination as

	either uncontrollable thought processes or as dangerous thought processes, such as "My worry can make me lose my mind". Fusion beliefs are also a form of metacognitive beliefs.
Metacognitive mode	means that the object of the thoughts is cognition itself. In MCT, the dialogue and exploration are about how the individual relates to their thoughts and thinking.
Object mode	means that the individual relates to thoughts as to perceptions of the external reality, as to the physical world. In MCT, the dialogue is conducted in metacognitive mode, i.e. the dialogue is focused on thoughts about the thoughts and about thinking.
OCD	Obsessive-compulsive disorder.
P-E-T-S	is an abbreviation for preparation, exposure, testing, summarizing in behavioral experiments in MCT. P-E-T-S means that a behavioral experiment is planned and carried out together with the client to test a certain metacognitive belief, and then summarized regarding the conclusions that can be drawn from the experiment.
Postponement of worry or rumination	is the act of noticing a trigger thought and further postponing the response to the negative thought until later, usually until a voluntary worry or thinking time.
PTSD	Post-traumatic stress disorder.
Reflexive adaptive process (RAP)	is the natural adaptation process that is assumed to be initiated after a traumatic event has occurred. RAP can be understood as a mental simulation of the trauma and its meaning in the form of spontaneous inner images and dreams. In the treatment of PTSD, CAS is believed to block the natural adaptation process that RAP constitutes.
Repetitive negative thinking (RNT)	is used as a collective term for worry and rumination.
Rumination	is a repetitive negative thought process and as such a CAS element. Rumination is often formulated as "Why ...?" It is a form of over-analysis of one's own well-being, one's own symptoms and the causes of the symptoms. Rumination can also apply to perceived injustice, or to memories of a course of events.

Self-regulatory executive function model, the S-REF model	The theoretical model on which MCT is based. The model describes cognition and information processing at three interacting levels, the meta-cognitive level, the online processing and the automatic level.
Situational attentional refocusing (SAR)	is an attentional technique in MCT. SAR aims to explicitly extend information processing to include things that are incompatible with the client's dysfunctional beliefs, for example in the treatment of social anxiety disorder or during later treatment phases of PTSD.
Spatial attention control exercise (SpACE)	is an attention exercise that aims to increase metacognitive awareness of thoughts, and that attention can be regulated flexibly independently of internal and external events.
Thought action fusion (TAF)	is a belief that the presence of an obsessive thought increases the risk that the individual will act on the thought against their will.
Thought event fusion (TEF)	is a belief that the presence of an obsession increases the risk of negative events or accidents occurring or having occurred.
Thought object fusion (TOF)	is a belief that negative thoughts and feelings can be transferred to physical objects and further on to other people.
Thought suppression	is actively trying to shut out a negative thought and keep it away from consciousness. It's a thought control strategy that usually has paradoxical effects.
Threat monitoring	is a form of biased attention where attention is directed to imagined external or internal threats and possible dangers. Threat monitoring is a coping strategy controlled by will and metacognition.
Trigger thought	is an association-driven, spontaneous thought that appears in consciousness. Trigger thoughts are to be understood as non-volitional.
Worry	is a negative, repetitive and future-oriented thought process. It's thinking about bad things that can happen. Worry is often formulated as "What if …" Worry is not the same as anxiety, which can instead be understood as an emotional, somatic experience. In the case of problems such as generalized anxiety, different forms of worry are described as type 1 worry and type 2 worry. Type 1 worry refers to worry about bad events that may occur. Type 2 worry refers to worry about worry.

Appendix 2: Measuring CAS and metacognition

This appendix presents instruments and methodologies that have been used in a research context and that can be used in the evaluation of treatment outcomes. In treatment evaluation, the instruments in this review can be used in combination with diagnosis-specific instruments to measure, for example, depression symptoms or different forms of anxiety symptoms in various psychological problems. In addition to instruments used in research that can be used in the evaluation of treatment outcomes, various process-measures have also been developed, instruments that are used repeatedly to guide the treatment process. The instruments developed to measure CAS and metacognition session by session, and which form an integral part of the treatment, have previously been described in Chapter 3.

Metacognitions questionnaires MCQ-65 and MCQ-30

In many of the studies mentioned in this book, the Metacognitions questionnaires MCQ-65 and MCQ-30 have been used to measure different dimensions of metacognition. These two forms are to be seen as "trait measures" of metacognition. The original instrument, the MCQ-65 (Cartwright-Hatton & Wells, 1997) consists of 65 items. The MCQ-30 is an abbreviated version with 30 items and shows corresponding psychometric properties (Wells & Cartwright-Hatton, 2004). A disadvantage of the MCQ-65 is the number of items and that it is more time-consuming, which is why the MCQ-30 was developed. The MCQ forms consist of the following five subscales: 1. Positive beliefs about worry (e.g. "worrying helps me cope"), 2. Negative beliefs about worry concerning uncontrollability and danger (e.g. "When I start worrying I cannot stop"), 3. Low cognitive confidence (e.g. "I have a poor memory"), 4. Need to control thoughts (e.g. "Not being able to control my thoughts is a sign of weakness"), 5. Cognitive self-consciousness (e.g. "I pay close attention to the way my mind works"). The internal consistency (Cronbach's alpha) of the subscales is high (0.72–0.89). Test retests over 5-week intervals range between 0.76 and 0.89 for the individual subscales. The subscales are positively correlated with *trait anxiety*, pathological anxiety, depressive symptoms, and OCD symptoms (Cartwright-Hatton & Wells, 1997; Gwilliam et al., 2004; Myers &

Wells, 2005; Wells & Cartwright-Hatton, 2004; Wells & Papageorgiou, 1998). In summary, the MCQ-65 shows good reliability and convergent, construct and discriminative validity. The subscales are sensitive to metacognitive therapy (Papageorgiou & Wells, 2000). The MCQ-30 exhibits similar psychometric properties to the MCQ-65 (Wells & Cartwright-Hatton, 2004). Cronbach's alpha for individual subscales ranges between 0.72 and 0.93.

Thought control questionnaire TCQ

TCQ (Wells & Davies, 1994) has been developed to measure individual differences in the use of strategies for dealing with unpleasant and intrusive thoughts. Thought suppression is not to be understood as a uniform construct but can be achieved in several different ways. The TCQ consists of 30 items, divided into five subscales. The five subscales are: 1. Distraction (e.g. "I do something that I enjoy"), 2. Social control (e.g. "I ask my friends if they have similar thoughts"), 3. Worry (e.g. "I focus on different negative thoughts"), 4. Punishment (e.g. "I punish myself for thinking the thought"), 5. Re-appraisal (e.g. "I try to reinterpret the thought"). The subscales "worry" and "punishment" have correlated positively with different symptom scales for emotional problems in various studies. Cronbach's alpha for the sub-scales ranges between 0.64 and 0.79. Test-retest correlations over a 6-week period were 0.72 for distraction, 0.79 for social control, 0.71 for anxiety, 0.64 for punishment, and 0.67 for re-evaluation (Wells & Davies, 1994). In terms of construct validity, the worry and punishment subscales are positively correlated with different measures of emotional problems and diagnoses such as OCD (Abramowitz et al., 2003; Amir et al., 1997).

Anxious thoughts inventory, AnTI

AnTI (Wells, 1994, 2000) has been designed as a multidimensional measure of worry, which aims to capture both basic worry themes and the difference between worry and negative appraisal of worry. Worry about non-cognitive events such as relationships and physical symptoms is referred to as type 1 anxiety. Worry about thoughts and worry about worry is called type 2 worry. The instrument consists of 22 items and is divided into three subscales: 1. Social worry (e.g. "I worry about doing or saying the wrong things when among strangers"), 2. Health worry (e.g. "I worry about having a heart attack or cancer"), 3. Meta-worry (e.g. "I worry that I cannot control my thoughts as well as I would like to"). In terms of psychometric properties, good reliability between subscales has been demonstrated with Cronbach's alpha between 0.75 and 0.84 and test-retest during 6 weeks between 0.76 and 0.84. Discriminative validity of AnTI has been established with diagnostic groups where type 2 worry has been significantly higher in patients with generalized anxiety compared to patients with panic disorder, social phobia and non-clinical control group.

Meta-Worry Questionnaire MWQ

AnTI combines the elements of uncontrollability and the danger of worry on the meta-worry scale. In addition, AnTI measures the frequency rather than the level of belief in meta-worry. The Meta-Worry Questionnaire MWQ (Wells, 2005a) was developed to specifically measure the danger aspect of meta-worry as well as to measure the frequency of meta-worry and the belief level. The instrument was developed to be able to test the metacognitive model in relation to generalized anxiety disorder according to DSM-IV. MWQ consists of 7 items that are supposed to reflect meta-beliefs about the worry as dangerous, such as "My worrying will escalate, and I'll cease to function". Cronbach's alpha for the frequency scale is 0.88 and for the belief scale 0.95. In terms of discriminative validity, MWQ differentiated between non-patients who nevertheless met criteria for GAD according to DSM-IV, and individuals assessed as somatically anxious and individuals without anxiety (Wells, 2005a).

Thought fusion instrument TFI

TFI was developed by Wells et al. (2001) and consists of 14 items. The instrument has been developed to measure fusion beliefs in the domains *of thought event fusion* (TEF), such as "My thoughts alone have the power to change the course of events", *thought action fusion* (TAF), such as "If I have thoughts of harming someone, I will act on them" and *thought object fusion* (TOF), for example, "My memories/thoughts can be passed into objects". These fusion beliefs are assumed to be relevant in the case formulation and treatment of OCD. The reliability, Cronbach's alpha, is good: 0.89. Positive correlations between TFI, MCQ, and measures of OCD symptoms have been found (Myers & Wells, 2005; Wells et al., 2001).

Positive beliefs about Rumination Scale PBRS and negative beliefs about Rumination Scale NBRS

Rumination is a central part of CAS and measuring metacognitive beliefs about rumination is therefore important. PBRS (Papageorgiou & Wells, 2001a) consists of nine items regarding positive metacognitive beliefs about rumination, such as "I need to ruminate about the bad things that happened in the past to make sense of them". Each item is rated along four scale steps from 1 (disagree) to 4 (agree very much). In terms of reliability, the internal consistency of PBRS was high, Cronbach's alpha 0.89 and the test-retest reliability over a 6-week period was 0.85.

NBRS (Papageorgiou et al., 2001) consists of two subscales, which aim to measure negative metacognitive beliefs about rumination. The first subscale, NBRS 1, consists of eight items regarding metacognitive beliefs about uncontrollability (e.g. "I cannot stop myself from ruminating") as well as the danger of rumination, e.g. "Ruminating makes me physically ill". The second subscale consists of five items regarding beliefs about the interpersonal and social consequences of rumination, for example "People will reject me if I ruminate". Each item is rated along four scale steps from 1 (disagree) to 4 (agree very much). In terms of reliability, Cronbach's alpha was 0.8 for NBRS 1 and 0.83 for NBRS 2.

Other instruments for measuring worry or rumination

There are also additional instruments and techniques for measuring worry, rumination and metacognition, which were not originally developed within an MCT context.

Penn State Worry Questionnaire PSWQ

PSWQ (Meyer et al., 1990) is one of the most internationally used instruments for measuring worry. The instrument consists of 16 items (e.g. "I'm always worrying about something"). The instrument shows good psychometric properties. For example, Behar et al. (2003) found that PSWQ is very well suited as a screening instrument for identifying GAD. In terms of reliability, the instrument has shown high internal consistency for both clinical and non-clinical groups (Molina & Borcovec, 1994). Cronbach's alpha has varied between 0.88 and 0.95. The PSWQ also shows good test-retest reliability, 0.74 to 0.92, in intervals between 2 and 10 weeks. The instrument has often been used in treatment studies and can also be used to evaluate treatment outcomes in GAD. In a review of *efficacy* for different psychological treatments for GAD and applying Jacobson and Truax (1991) criteria for clinical significance, Fisher (2006) calculated the *reliable change index* (RCI) to be 7 for PSWQ and the cutoff value to ≤ 47. For more in-depth reasoning about cutoff values and the qualities of the instrument, see Startup and Erickson (2006). PSWQ has also shown sensitivity to therapeutic change over both 6 and 12 weeks of therapeutic interventions for GAD (Borkovec & Costello, 1993).

Generalized Anxiety Disorder Questionnaire-IV, GAD-Q-IV

GAD-Q-IV (Newman et al., 2002) has been developed for initial screening of the presence or absence of the diagnosis of GAD according to DSM-IV criteria. The instrument consists of nine items about anxiety and physical symptoms of anxiety (e.g. "Do you experience excessive worry?" or "Do you worry excessively or uncontrollably about minor things such as being late for an appointment, minor repairs, homework, etc?") A cutoff value of 5.7 points (83 percent sensitivity and 89 percent specificity) on GAD-Q-IV has been shown to indicate the presence of a diagnosis of GAD. According to the authors, those who want increased certainty that only individuals with

GAD are included in a sample, can instead choose a higher cutoff value of 9. In terms of reliability, GAD-Q-IV has shown good internal consistency, Cronbach's alpha 0.84. Test-retest reliability is according to Newman et al. (2002) 0.81 over a period of 2 weeks.

Rumination Response Scale RRS 10

RRS 10 (Treynor et al., 2003) consists of ten items, divided into the two sub-scales: Reflection (e.g. "I write down my thoughts and analyze them") and Brooding (e.g. "Why do I have problems that other people don't?"). RRS 10 is a shortened version of the original RRS with 22 items. In RRS 10, items that have been shown to overlap with depression symptoms have been removed. The instruments have been developed in light of the fact that rumination has been shown as an important factor in depression. Parola et al. (2017) found among outpatients with a depression diagnosis (n = 100) that RRS 10 showed acceptable reliability, Cronbach's alpha between 0.74 and 0.83. As expected in that study, rumination was associated with depression severity.

Instantaneous measurements of metacognition and CAS, Experience Sampling methods or Ecological Momentary Assessment

Measurements with instruments like those reviewed here give retrospective data. To counter sources of error associated with retrospective data, so-called *recall bias*, newer methods have been developed where more instantaneous and repeated self-assessments can be made, for example, with a smartphone. Experience Sampling or Ecological Momentary Assessment are techniques designed to identify individuals' behaviors, thoughts or feelings in real time and in the natural environments of the individual. For example, in studies by Aadahl et al. (2021), Hallard et al. (2021), Kubiak et al. (2014) and Thielsh et al. (2015), Experience Sampling was used to measure CAS and metacognition.

References

Aadahl, V., Wells, A., Hallard, R. & Pratt, D. (2021). Metacognitive beliefs and suicidal ideation: An experience sampling study. *International Journal of Environmental Research and Public Health*, 18(23), 12336.

Abramowitz, J.S., Whiteside, S., Kalsy, S.A. & Tolin, D.F. (2003). Thought control strategies in obsessive-compulsive disorder: A replication and extension. *Behaviour Research and Therapy*, 41(5), 529–540.

Af Winklerfelt Hammarberg, S., Toth-Pal, E., Jansson-Fröjmark, M., Lundgren, T., Westman, J. & Bohman, B. (2023). Intolerance-of-uncertainty therapy versus metacognitive therapy for generalized anxiety disorder in primary health care: A randomized controlled pilot trial. *PloS one*, 18(6), e0287171.

Allen, A., Kannis-Dymand, L. & Katsikitis, M. (2017). Problematic internet pornography use: The role of craving, desire thinking, and metacognition. *Addictive Behaviors*, 70, 65–71.

Allott, R., Wells, A., Morrison, A.P. & Walker, R. (2005). Distress in Parkinson's disease: Contributions of disease factors and metacognitive style. *British Journal of Psychiatry*, 187(2), 182–183.

American Psychological Association (2017). Ethical principles of psychologists and code of conduct (2002). Amended effective June 1, 2010, and January 2017.

Amir, N., Cashman, L. & Foa, E.B. (1997). Strategies of thought control in obsessive-compulsive disorder. *Behaviour Research and Therapy*, 35(8), 775–777.

Anderson, R., Capobianco, L., Fisher, P., Reeves, D., Heal, C., ... & Wells, A. (2019). Testing relationships between metacognitive beliefs, anxiety and depression in cardiac and cancer patients: Are they transdiagnostic? *Journal of Psychosomatic Research*, 124, 109738.

Andersson, E., Aspvall, K., Schettini, G., Kraepelien, M., Särnholm, J., Wergeland, G.J. & Öst, L.G. (2024). Efficacy of metacognitive interventions for psychiatric disorders: A systematic review and meta-analysis. *Cognitive Behaviour Therapy*, 1–27. Advance online publication.

Austin, S.F., Mors, O., Nordentoft, M., Hjorthøj, C.R., Secher, R.G., ... & Wells, A. (2014). Schizophrenia and metacognition: An investigation of course of illness and metacognitive beliefs within a first episode psychosis. *Cognitive Therapy and Research*, 39, 61–69.

Aydin, O., Balıkçı, K., Çökmüs, F.P. & Ünal Aydin, P. (2019). The evaluation of metacognitive beliefs and emotion recognition in panic disorder and generalized anxiety disorder: Effects on symptoms and comparison with healthy control. *Nordic Journal of Psychiatry*, 73(4–5), 293–301.

Bailey, R. & Wells, A. (2014). Metacognitive therapy in the treatment of hypochondriasis: A systematic case series. *Cognitive Therapy and Research*, 38, 541–550.

Bailey, R. & Wells, A. (2015). Metacognitive beliefs moderate the relationship between catastrophic misinterpretation and health anxiety. *Journal of Anxiety Disorders*, 34, 8–14.

Bailey, R. & Wells, A. (2016). The contribution of metacognitive beliefs and dysfunctional illness beliefs in predicting health anxiety: An evaluation of the metacognitive versus the cognitive models. *Clinical Psychologist*, 20, 129–137.

Bailey, R. & Wells, A. (2024). Feasibility and preliminary efficacy of metacognitive therapy for health anxiety: A pilot RCT. *Journal of Affective Disorders Reports*, (16) 2024.

Baker, H.J., Lawrence, P.J., Karalus, J., Creswell, C. & Waite, P. (2021). The effectiveness of psychological therapies for anxiety disorders in adolescents: A meta-analysis. *Clinical Child and Family Psychology Review*, 24(4), 765–782.

Bakker, G.M. (2019). A new conception and subsequent taxonomy of clinical psychological problems. *BMC Psychology*, 7(1), 46.

Bakker, G.M. (2022). Psychotherapy outcome research: Implications of a new clinical taxonomy. *Clinical Psychology & Psychotherapy*, 29(1), 178–199.

Bar-Haim, Y., Lamy, D., Pergamin, L., Bakermans-Kranenburg, M.J. & van IJzendoorn, M.H. (2007). Threat related attentional bias in anxious and nonanxious individuals: A meta-analytic study. *Psychological Bulletin*, 133, 1–24.

Barrett, L.F. (2017). The theory of constructed emotion: An active inference account of interoception and categorization. *Social Cognitive and Affective Neuroscience*, 12(1), 1–23.

Batmaz, S., Altinoz, A.E. & Sonkurt, H.O. (2021). Cognitive attentional syndrome and metacognitive beliefs as potential treatment targets for metacognitive therapy in bipolar disorder. *World Journal of Psychiatry*, 11(9), 589–604.

Beck, A.T., Rush, A.J., Shaw, B.F. & Emery, G. (1979). *Cognitive therapy of depression*. Guilford Press.

Beck, J. (2011). *Cognitive behavior therapy, basics and beyond* (2nd ed.). Guilford.

Behar, E., Alcaine, O., Zuellig, A.R. & Borkovec, T.D. (2003). Screening for generalized anxiety disorder using the Penn State Worry Questionnaire: A receiver operating characteristic analysis. *Journal of Behavior Therapy and Experimental Psychiatry*, 34, 25–43.

Bennett, H. & Wells, A. (2010). Metacognition, memory disorganization and rumination in posttraumatic stress symptoms. *Journal of Anxiety Disorders*, 24, 318–325.

Bianchi, R., Boffy, C., Hingray, C., Truchot, D. & Laurent, E. (2013). Comparative sympto-matology of burnout and depression. *Journal of Health Psychology*, 18(6), 782–787.

Bianchi, R., Schonfeld, I.S. & Laurent, E. (2015). Burnout-depression overlap: A review. *Clinical Psychology Review*, 36, 28–41.

Blackburn, I.-M., James, I.A., Milne, D.L., Baker, C., Standart, S., ... & Reichelt, F. K. (2001). The revised cognitive therapy scale (CTS-R): Psychometric properties. *Behavioural and Cognitive Psychotherapy*, 29(4), 431–446.

Boettcher, H., Brake, C.A. & Barlow, D.H. (2016). Origins and outlook of interoceptive exposure. *Journal of Behavior Therapy and Experimental Psychiatry*, 53, 41–51.

Bonner, J., Allen, A., Katsikitis, M., Love, S. & Kannis-Dymand, L. (2022). Metacognition, desire thinking and craving in problematic video game use. *Journal of Technology in Behavioral Science*, 7(4), 532–546.

Borkovec, T.D. & Costello, E. (1993). Efficacy of applied relaxation and cognitive-behavioral therapy in the treatment of generalized anxiety disorder. *Journal of Consulting and Clinical Psychology*, 61(4), 611–619.

Borkovec, T.D., Robinson, E., Pruzinsky, T. & DePree, J.A. (1983). Preliminary exploration of worry: Some characteristics and processes. *Behaviour Research and Therapy*, 21(1), 9–16.

Boschen, M.J. (2007). Reconceptualizing emetophobia: A cognitive-behavioral formulation and research agenda. *Journal of Anxiety Disorders*, 21(3), 407–419.

Bowlby, J. (1969). *Attachment and loss: Vol. 1: Attachment*. Basic Books.

Breslau, N. (2002). Epidemiologic studies of trauma, posttraumatic stress disorder, and other psychiatric disorders. *Canadian Journal of Psychiatry. Revue Canadienne de Psychiatrie*, 47(10), 923–929.

Bright, M., Parker, S., French, P., Fowler, D., Gumley, A., ... & Wells, A. (2018). Metacognitive beliefs as psychological predictors of social functioning: An investigation with young people at risk of psychosis. *Psychiatry Research*, 262, 520–526.

British Psychological Society (2021). *Code of Ethics and conduct*. https://explore.bps. org.uk/content/report-guideline/bpsrep.2021.inf94. Downloaded June 10, 2024).

Brown, R.L., Wood, A., Carter, J.D. & Kannis-Dymand, L. (2022). The metacognitive model of post-traumatic stress disorder and metacognitive therapy for post-traumatic stress disorder: A systematic review. *Clinical Psychology & Psychotherapy*, 29(1), 131–146.

Buysse, D.J. (2013). Insomnia. *Journal of the American Medical Association*, 309 (7), 706–716.

Caldarone, F., Gebhardt, P., Hoeper, M.M., Olsson, K.M., Fuge, J., ... & Heitland, I. (2022). Metacognitions in patients with frequent mental disorders after diagnosis of pulmonary arterial hypertension. *Frontiers in Psychiatry*, 13, 812812.

Callesen, P., Capobianco, L., Heal, C., Juul, C., Find Nielsen, S. & Wells, A. (2019). A preliminary evaluation of transdiagnostic group metacognitive therapy in a mixed psychological disorder sample. *Frontiers in Psychology*, 10, 1341.

Callesen, P., Reeves, D., Heal, C. & Wells, A. (2020a). Metacognitive therapy versus cognitive behaviour therapy in adults with major depression: A parallel single-blind randomised trial. *Scientific Reports*, 10, 7878.

Callesen, P., Lunde Pedersen, M., Koch Andersen, C. & Wells, A. (2020b). Metacognitive therapy for bipolar II disorder: A single case series study. *Neurology, Psychiatry and Brain Research*, 38, 107–113.

Cano-López, J.B., García-Sancho, E., Fernández-Castilla, B. & Salguero, J.M. (2021). Empirical evidence of the metacognitive model of rumination and depression in clinical and nonclinical samples: A systematic review and meta-analysis. *Cognitive Therapy and Research*, 46, 367–392.

Capobianco, L. & Nordahl, H. (2023). A brief history of metacognitive therapy: From cognitive science to clinical practice. *Cognitive and Behavioral Practice*, 30(1), 45–54.

Carpenter, J.K., Andrews, L.A., Witcraft, S.M., Powers, M.B., Smits, J.A.J. & Hofmann, S.G. (2018). Cognitive behavioral therapy for anxiety and related disorders: A meta-analysis of randomized placebo-controlled trials. *Depression and Anxiety*, 35(6), 502–514.

Carter, J., Helliwell, E., Jordan, J., Woolcock, C., Bell, C. & Gilbert, C. (2022a). Group metacognitive therapy for obsessive-compulsive disorder in a routine clinical setting: An open trial. *Behaviour Change*, 1–16.

Carter, J.D., Jordan, J., McIntosh, V.V., Frampton, C.M., Lacey, C., ... & Mulder, R.T. (2022b). Long-term efficacy of metacognitive therapy and cognitive behaviour therapy for depression. *The Australian and New Zealand Journal of Psychiatry*, 56(2), 137–143.

Cartwright-Hatton, S. & Wells, A. (1997). Beliefs about worry and intrusions: The Meta-Cognitions Questionnaire and its correlates. *Journal of Anxiety Disorders*, 11(3), 279–296.

Caselli, G., Ferretti, C., Leoni, M., Rebecchi, D., Rovetto, F. & Spada, M.M. (2010). Rumination as a predictor of drinking behaviour in alcohol abusers: A prospective study. *Addiction*, 105(6), 1041–1048.

Caselli, G., Gemelli, A., Ferrari, C., Beltrami, D., Offredi, A., ... & Spada, M.M. (2021). The effect of desire thinking on facilitating beliefs in alcohol use disorder: An experimental investigation. *Clinical Psychology & Psychotherapy*, 28(2), 355–363.

Caselli, G., Martino, F., Spada, M.M. & Wells, A. (2018). Metacognitive therapy for alcohol use disorder: A systematic case series. *Frontiers in Psychology*, 9, 2619.

Caselli, G., Offredi, A., Martino, F., Varalli, D., Ruggiero, G.M., ... & Wells, A. (2017). Metacognitive beliefs and rumination as predictors of anger: A prospective study. *Aggressive Behavior*, 43(5), 421–429.

Caselli, G., Soliani, M. & Spada, M.M. (2013). The effect of desire thinking on craving: An experimental investigation. *Psychology of Addictive Behaviors*, 27(1), 301–306.

Caselli, G. & Spada, M.M. (2010). Metacognitions in desire thinking: A preliminary investigation. *Behavioural and Cognitive Psychotherapy*, 38(5), 629–637.

Caselli, G. & Spada, M.M. (2015). Desire thinking: What is it and what drives it? *Addictive Behaviors*, 44, 71–79.

Cavicchioli, M. & Maffei, C. (2022). Rumination as a widespread emotion-based cognitive vulnerability in borderline personality disorder: A meta-analytic review. *Journal of Clinical Psychology*, 78(6), 989–1008.

Chen, J.H., Spada, M.M., Ling, H., Tong, K.K. & Wu, A.M.S. (2024). Desire thinking about gambling: Assessment and associations with gambling disorder and responsible gambling among Chinese gamblers. *Journal of Gambling Studies*, 40 (3), 1423–1438.

Chen, J., Tan, Y., Cheng, X., Peng, Z., Qin, C., ... & Lei, W. (2021). Maladaptive metacognitive beliefs mediated the effect of intolerance of uncertainty on depression. *Clinical Psychology & Psychotherapy*, 28(6), 1525–1534.

Cisler, J.M. & Koster, E.H. (2010). Mechanisms of attentional bias towards threat in anxiety disorders: An integrative review. *Clinical Psychology Review*, 30, 203–216.

Clancy, F., Prestwich, A., Caperon, L. & O'Connor, D.B. (2016). Perseverative cognition and health behaviors: A systematic review and meta-analysis. *Frontiers in Human Neuroscience*, 10, 534.

Clancy, F., Prestwich, A., Caperon, L., Tsipa, A. & O'Connor, D.B. (2020). The association between worry and rumination with sleep in non-clinical populations: A systematic review and meta-analysis. *Health Psychology Review*, 14(4), 427–448.

Clark, D.M. (1986). A cognitive approach to panic. *Behaviour Research and Therapy*, 24, 461–470.

Clark, D.M. & Wells, A. (1995). A cognitive model of social phobia. In: R. Heimberg, M. Liebowitz, D.A. Hope & F.R. Schneier (eds.), *Social phobia: Diagnosis, assessment and treatment*. Guilford Press.

Coleman, S.E., Dunlop, B.J., Hartley, S. & Taylor, P.J. (2022). The relationship between rumination and NSSI: A systematic review and meta-analysis. *The British Journal of Clinical Psychology*, 61(2), 405–443.

Conway, C.C., Forbes, M.K., Forbush, K.T., Fried, E.I., Hallquist, M.N., ... & Eaton, N.R. (2019). A hierarchical taxonomy of psychopathology can transform mental health research. *Perspectives on Psychological Science: A Journal of the Association for Psychological Science*, 14(3), 419–436.

Conway, C.C., Forbes, M.K., South, S.C. & HiTOP Consortium (2022). A hierarchical taxonomy of psychopathology (HiTOP) primer for mental health researchers. *Clinical Psychological Science: A Journal of the Association for Psychological Science*, 10(2), 236–258.

Cowen, P.J. & Browning, M. (2015). What has serotonin to do with depression? *World Psychiatry: Official Journal of the World Psychiatric Association (WPA)*, 14(2), 158–160.

Craske, M.G., Treanor, M., Conway, C.C., Zbozinek, T. & Vervliet, B. (2014). Maximizing exposure therapy: An inhibitory learning approach. *Behaviour Research and Therapy*, 58, 10–23.

Cucchi, M., Bottelli, V., Cavadini, D., Ricci, L., Conca, V., ... & Smeraldi, E. (2012). An explorative study on metacognition in obsessive-compulsive disorder and panic disorder. *Comprehensive Psychiatry*, 53(5), 546–553.

Cuijpers, P., Karyotaki, E., Ciharova, M., Miguel, C., Noma, H. & Furukawa, T.A. (2021). The effects of psychotherapies for depression on response, remission, reliable change, and deterioration: A meta-analysis. *Acta Psychiatrica Scandinavica*, 144(3), 288–299.

Dalgleish, T., Black, M., Johnston, D. & Bevan, A. (2020). Transdiagnostic approaches to mental health problems: Current status and future directions. *Journal of Consulting and Clinical Psychology*, 88(3), 179–195.

Dammen, T., Papageorgiou, C. & Wells, A. (2015). An open trial of group metacognitive therapy for depression in Norway. *Nordic Journal of Psychiatry*, 69(2), 126–131.

Dammen, T., Papageorgiou, C. & Wells, A. (2016). A two year follow up study of group metacognitive therapy for depression in Norway. *Journal of Depression and Anxiety*, 5, 227.

Davey, G.C.L. & Wells, A. (eds.) (2006). *Worry and its psychological disorders: Theory, assessment and treatment*. Wiley.

De Dominicis, S., Troen, M.L. & Callesen, P. (2021). Metacognitive therapy for work-related stress: A feasibility study. *Frontiers in Psychiatry*, 12, 668245.

Deguchi, A., Masuya, J., Naruse, M., Morishita, C., Higashiyama, M., ... & Ichiki, M. (2021). Rumination mediates the effects of childhood maltreatment and trait anxiety on depression in non-clinical adult volunteers. *Neuropsychiatric Disease and Treatment*, 17, 3439–3445.

Deleurme, K.A., Parkinson, S.A. & Penney, A.M. (2022). Generalized anxiety disorder: Does the emotion dysregulation model predict symptoms beyond the metacognitive model? *Journal of Rational-Emotive and Cognitive-Behavior Therapy: RET*, 1–17. Advance online publication.

Devynck, F., Rousseau, A. & Romo, L. (2019). Does repetitive negative thinking influence alcohol use? A systematic review of the literature. *Frontiers in Psychology*, 10, 1482.

Dodd, R., Fisher, P.L., Makin, S., Moore, P. & Cherry, M.G. (2021). The association between maladaptive metacognitive beliefs and emotional distress in people living with amyotrophic lateral sclerosis. *Frontiers in Psychology*, 12, 609068.

Eisma, M.C., Boelen, P.A., Schut, H.A. & Stroebe, M.S. (2017). Does worry affect adjustment to bereavement? A longitudinal investigation. *Anxiety, Stress, and Coping*, 30(3), 243–252.

Eisma, M.C., de Lang, T.A. & Boelen, P.A. (2020). How thinking hurts: Rumination, worry, and avoidance processes in adjustment to bereavement. *Clinical Psychology & Psychotherapy*, 27(4), 548–558.

Eisma, M.C., Franzen, M., Paauw, M., Bleeker, A. & Aan Het Rot, M. (2022). Rumination, worry and negative and positive affect in prolonged grief: A daily diary study. *Clinical Psychology & Psychotherapy*, 29(1), 299–312.

Esbjørn, B.H., Lønfeldt, N.N., Nielsen, S.K., Reinholdt-Dunne, M.L., Sømhovd, M. J. & Cartwright-Hatton, S. (2015). Meta-worry, worry, and anxiety in children and adolescents: Relationships and interactions. *Journal of Clinical Child & Adolescent Psychology*, 44(1), 145–156.

Esbjørn, B.H., Normann, N., Christiansen, B.M. & Reinholdt-Dunne, M.L. (2018). The efficacy of group metacognitive therapy for children (MCT-c) with generalized anxiety disorder: An open trial. *Journal of Anxiety Disorders*, 53, 16–21.

Esbjørn, B.H., Normann, N. & Reinholdt-Dunne, M.L. (2016). *Metakognitiv terapi til børn med angst* [Metacognitive therapy for children with anxiety]. Akademisk Vorlag.

Espeleta, H.C., Taylor, D.L., Kraft, J.D. & Grant, D.M. (2021). Child maltreatment and cognitive vulnerabilities: Examining the link to posttraumatic stress symptoms. *Journal of American College Health*, 69(7), 759–766.

Exner, C., Kleiman, A., Haberkamp, A., Hansmeier, J., Milde, C. & Glombiewski, J.A. (2024). Metacognitive therapy versus exposure and response prevention for obsessive-compulsive disorder: A non-inferiority randomized control trial. *Journal of Anxiety Disorders*, 104, 102873.

Fairburn, C.G. (2008). *Cognitive behavior therapy and eating disorders*. Guilford Press.

Fearn, M., Marino, C., Spada, M.M. & Kolubinski, D.C. (2022). Self-critical rumination and associated metacognitions as mediators of the relationship between perfectionism and self-esteem. *Journal of Rational-Emotive and Cognitive Behavior Therapy: RET*, 40(1), 155–174.

Fergus, T.A. & Wheless, N.E. (2018). The attention training technique causally reduces self-focus following worry provocation and reduces cognitive anxiety among self-focused individuals. *Journal of Behavior Therapy and Experimental Psychiatry*, 61, 66–71.

Fernie, B.A., Spada, M.M., Ray Chaudhuri, K., Klingelhoefer, L. & Brown, R.G. (2015). Thinking about motor fluctuations: An examination of metacognitions in Parkinson's disease. *Journal of Psychosomatic Research*, 79(6), 669–673.

Fisher, P.L. (2006). The efficacy of psychological treatments for generalized anxiety disorder? Predictors of treatment outcome. In: G.C.L. Davey & A. Wells (eds.), *Worry and its psychological disorders: Theory, assessment and treatment* (pp. 359–377). Wiley.

Fisher, P.L., Byrne, A., Fairburn, L., Ullmer, H., Abbey, G. & Salmon, P. (2019). Brief metacognitive therapy for emotional distress in adult cancer survivors. *Frontiers in Psychology*, 10, 162.

Fisher, P.L., Byrne, A. & Salmon, P. (2017). Metacognitive therapy for emotional distress in adult cancer survivors: A case series. *Cognitive Therapy and Research*, 41(6), 891–901.

Fisher, P.L., McNicol, K., Young, B., Smith, E. & Salmon P. (2015). Alleviating emotional distress in adolescent and young adult cancer survivors: An open trial of meta-cognitive therapy. *Journal of Adolescent and Young Adult Oncology*, 4 (2), 64–69.

Fisher, P. & Wells, A. (2009). *Metacognitive therapy: Distinctive features*. Routledge.

Foa, E.B., Hembree, E.A. & Rothbaum, B.O. (2007). *Prolonged exposure therapy for PTSD, emotional processing of traumatic experiences: Therapist guide*. Oxford University Press.

Freeman, D., Dunn, G., Startup, H., Pugh, K., Cordwell, J., ... & Kingdon, D. (2015). Effects of cognitive behaviour therapy for worry on persecutory delusions in patients with psychosis (WIT): A parallel, single-blind, randomised controlled trial with a mediation analysis. *The Lancet Psychiatry*, 2(4), 305–313.

Freeman, D. & Garety, P. (2014). Advances in understanding and treating persecutory delusions: A review. *Social Psychiatry and Psychiatric Epidemiology*, 49(8), 1179–1189.

Freeston, M., Rheaume, J., Letarte, H., Dugas, M. & Ladouceur, R. (1994). Why do people worry? *Personality and Individual Differences*, 17, 791–802.

Frøjd, L.A., Papageorgiou, C., Munkhaugen, J., Moum, T., Sverre, E., ... & Dammen, T. (2022). Worry and rumination predict insomnia in patients with coronary heart disease: A cross-sectional study with long-term follow-up. *Journal of Clinical Sleep Medicine: JCSM: Official Publication of the American Academy of Sleep Medicine*, 18(3), 779–787.

Galatzer-Levy, I.R., Huang, S.H. & Bonanno, G.A. (2018). Trajectories of resilience and dysfunction following potential trauma: A review and statistical evaluation. *Clinical Psychology Review*, 63, 41–55.

Galbiati, A., Giora, E., Sarasso, S., Zucconi, M. & Ferini-Strambi, L. (2018). Repetitive thought is associated with both subjectively and objectively recorded polysomnographic indices of disrupted sleep in insomnia disorder. *Sleep Medicine*, 45, 55–61.

Galbiati, A., Sforza, M., Scarpellino, A., Salibba, A., Leitner, C., ... & Castronovo, V. (2021). "Thinking about thinking" in insomnia disorder: The effect of cognitive-behavioral therapy for insomnia on sleep-related metacognition. *Frontiers in Psychology*, 12, 705112.

Gavric, D., Moscovitch, D.A., Rowa, K. & McCabe, R.E. (2017). Post-event processing in social anxiety disorder: Examining the mediating roles of positive metacognitive beliefs and perceptions of performance. *Behaviour Research and Therapy*, 91, 1–12.

Gilbert, P. (2010). *Compassion focused therapy: Distinctive features*. CBT distinctive features series. Routledge.

Glombiewski, J.A., Hansmeier, J., Haberkamp, A., Rief, W. & Exner, C. (2021). Metacognitive therapy versus exposure and response prevention for obsessive-compulsive disorder: A pilot randomized trial. *Journal of Obsessive-Compulsive and Related Disorders*, 30, 100650.

Goldsmith, A.A., Tran, G.Q., Smith, J.P. & Howe, S.R. (2009). Alcohol expectancies and drinking motives in college drinkers: Mediating effects on the relationship between generalized anxiety and heavy drinking in negative-affect situations. *Addictive Behaviors*, 34(6–7), 505–513.

Gutierrez, R., Hirani, T., Curtis, L. & Ludlow, A.K. (2020). Metacognitive beliefs mediate the relationship between anxiety sensitivity and traits of obsessive-compulsive symptoms. *BMC Psychology*, 8(1), 40.

Gwilliam, P., Wells, A. & Cartwright-Hatton, S. (2004). Does meta-cognition or responsibility predict obsessive-compulsive symptoms? A test of the metacognitive model. *Clinical Psychology & Psychotherapy*, 11(2), 137–144.

Hagen, R., Havnen, A., Hjemdal, O., Kennair, L., Ryum, T. & Solem, S. (2020). Protective and vulnerability factors in self-esteem: The role of metacognitions, brooding, and resilience. *Frontiers in Psychology*, 11, 1447.

Hagen, R., Hjemdal, O., Solem, S., Kennair, L.E., Nordahl, H.M., ... & Wells, A. (2017). Metacognitive therapy for depression in adults: A waiting list randomized controlled trial with six months follow-up. *Frontiers in Psychology*, 24(8), 31.

Halaj, A., Strauss, A.Y., Zalaznik, D., Fradkin, I., Zlotnick, E., Andersson, G., Ebert, D.D. & Huppert, J.D. (2023). Examining the relationship between cognitive factors and insight in panic disorder before and during treatment. *Cognitive Behavioral Therapy*, 52 (4), 331–346.

Hallard, R.I., Wells, A., Aadahl, V., Emsley, R. & Pratt, D. (2021). Metacognition, rumination and suicidal ideation: An experience sampling test of the self-regulatory executive function model. *Psychiatry Research*, 303, 114083.

Hames, J.L., Ribeiro, J.D., Smith, A.R. & Joiner, T.E. Jr. (2012). An urge to jump affirms the urge to live: An empirical examination of the high place phenomenon. *Journal of Affective Disorders*, 136(3), 1114–1120.

Hammersmark, A.T., Hjemdal, O., Hannisdal, M., Lending, H.D., Reme, S.E., Hodne, K., Osnes, K., Gjengedal, R. & Johnson, S.U. (2024) Metacognitive therapy for generalized anxiety disorders in group: A case study. *Journal of Clinical Psychology*, 80(4) 884–899.

Hansmeier, J., Haberkamp, A., Glombiewski, J.A. & Exner, C. (2021). Metacognitive change during exposure and metacognitive therapy in obsessive-compulsive disorder. *Frontiers of Psychiatry*, 3(12), 722782.

Harmer, B., Lee, S., Duong, T. & Saadabadi, A. (2021). Suicidal ideation. In *StatPearls*. StatPearls Publishing.

Hartley, S., Haddock, G., Vasconcelos e Sa, D., Emsley, R. & Barrowclough, C. (2014). An experience sampling study of worry and rumination in psychosis. *Psychological Medicine*, 44(8), 1605–1614.

Hartley, S., Haddock, G., Vasconcelos e Sa, D., Emsley, R. & Barrowclough, C. (2015). The influence of thought control on the experience of persecutory delusions and auditory hallucinations in daily life. *Behaviour Research and Therapy*, 65, 1–4.

Haseth, S., Solem, S., Sørø, G.B., Bjørnstad, E., Grøtte, T. & Fisher, P. (2019). Group metacognitive therapy for generalized anxiety disorder: A pilot feasibility trial. *Frontiers in Psychology*, 10, 290.

Havnen, A., Anyan, F. & Nordahl, H. (2024) Metacognitive strategies mediate the association between metacognitive beliefs and perceived quality of life. *Scandinavian Journal of Psychology*, 65(4), 656–664.

Hayes, S.C., Strosahl, K.D. & Wilson, K.G. (1999). *Acceptance and commitment therapy: An experiential approach to behavior change*. Guilford Press.

Healy, D. (2015). Serotonin and depression. *BMJ (Clinical Research Ed.)*, 350, h1771.

Heffer-Rahn, P. & Fisher, P.L. (2018). The clinical utility of metacognitive beliefs and processes in emotional distress in people with multiple sclerosis. *Journal of Psychosomatic Research*, 104, 88–94.

Hjemdal, O., Solem, S., Hagen, R., Ottesen Kennair, L.E., Nordahl, H.M. & Wells, A. (2019). A randomized controlled trial of metacognitive therapy for depression: Analysis of 1-year follow-up. *Frontiers in Psychology*, 10, 1842.

Holmes, E.A., Ghaderi, A., Harmer, C.J., Ramchandani, P.G., Cuijpers, P., ... & Craske, M.G. (2018). The Lancet Psychiatry Commission on psychological treatments research in tomorrow's science. *The Lancet Psychiatry*, 5(3), 237–286.

Holt-Lunstad, J., Smith, T.B., Baker, M., Harris, T. & Stephenson, D. (2015). Loneliness and social isolation as risk factors for mortality: A meta-analytic review. *Perspectives on Psychological Science*, 10(2), 227–237.

Horváth, D., Kovács-Tóth, B., Oláh, B. & Fekete, Z. (2024). Trends in the dose–response relationship between adverse childhood experiences and maladaptive metacognitive beliefs: a cross-sectional study. *Comprehensive Psychiatry*, 132, 152489.

Huntley, C., Young, B., Tudur Smith, C., Jha, V. & Fisher, P. (2022). Testing times: The association of intolerance of uncertainty and metacognitive beliefs to test anxiety in college students. *BMC Psychology*, 10(1), 6.

Hutton, P., Morrison, A.P., Wardle, M. & Wells, A. (2014). Metacognitive therapy in treatment-resistant psychosis: A multiple-baseline study. *Behavioural and Cognitive Psychotherapy*, 42(2), 166–185.

Ingram, R.E. (1990). Self-focused attention in clinical disorders: Review and a conceptual model. *Psychological Bulletin*, 107(2), 156–176.

Jacobsen, H.B., Aasvik, J.K., Borchgrevink, P.C., Landrø, N.I. & Stiles, T.C. (2016). Metacognitions are associated with subjective memory problems in individuals on sick leave due to chronic fatigue. *Frontiers in Psychology*, 7, 729.

Jacobson, N.S. & Truax, P. (1991). Clinical significance: A statistical approach to defining meaningful change in psychotherapy research. *Journal of Consulting and Clinical Psychology*, 59, 12–19.

Jannati, Y., Nia, H.S., Froelicher, E.S., Goudarzian, A.H. & Yaghoobzadeh, A. (2020). Self-blame attributions of patients: A systematic review study. *Central Asian Journal of Global Health*, 9(1), e419.

Jericho, B., Luo, A. & Berle, D. (2022). Trauma-focused psychotherapies for post-traumatic stress disorder: A systematic review and network meta-analysis. *Acta Psychiatrica Scandinavica*, 145(2), 132–155.

Johnsen, T.J. & Friborg, O. (2015). The effects of cognitive behavioral therapy as an anti- depressive treatment is falling: A meta-analysis. *Psychological Bulletin*, 141 (4), 747–768.

Johnson, S.U., Hoffart, A., Nordahl, H.M. & Wampold, B.E. (2017). Metacognitive therapy versus disorder-specific CBT for comorbid anxiety disorders: A randomized controlled trial. *Journal of Anxiety Disorders*, 50, 103–112.

Jordan, J., Carter, J.D., McIntosh, V.V.W., Fernando, K., Frampton, C.M., ... & Joyce, P.R. (2014). Metacognitive therapy versus cognitive behavioural therapy for depression: A randomized pilot study. *Australian and New Zealand Journal of Psychiatry*, 48(10), 932–943.

Juul, C. (2019). *Stress dig sund, et opgør med stressmyterne* [Stress yourself to health, challenging the myths of stress]. Saxo.

Kamboj, S.K., Langhoff, C., Pajak, R., Zhu, A., Chevalier, A. & Watson, S. (2015). Bowel and bladder-control anxiety: A preliminary description of a viscerally-centered phobic syndrome. *Behavioural and Cognitive Psychotherapy*, 43(2), 142–157.

Kannis-Dymand, L., Hughes, E., Mulgrew, K., Carter, J.D. & Love, S. (2020). Examining the roles of metacognitive beliefs and maladaptive aspects of perfectionism in depression and anxiety. *Behavioural and Cognitive Psychotherapy*, 48 (4), 442–453.

Keen, E., Kangas, M. & Gilchrist, P.T. (2022). A systematic review evaluating metacognitive beliefs in health anxiety and somatic distress. *British Journal of Health Psychology*, 27(4), 1398–1422.

Keller, A., Litzelman, K., Wisk, L.E., Maddox, T., Cheng, E.R., … & Witt, W.P. (2012). Does the perception that stress affects health matter? The association with health and mortality. *Health Psychology: Official Journal of the Division of Health Psychology, American Psychology Association*, 31(5), 677–684.

Kennair, L., Solem, S., Hagen, R., Havnen, A., Nysaeter, T.E. & Hjemdal, O. (2021). Change in personality traits and facets (Revised NEO Personality Inventory) following metacognitive therapy or cognitive behaviour therapy for generalized anxiety disorder: Results from a randomized controlled trial. *Clinical Psychology & Psychotherapy*, 28(4), 872–881.

Kessler, R.C., Chiu, W.T., Jin, R., Ruscio, A.M., Shear, K. & Walters, E.E. (2006). The epidemiology of panic attacks, panic disorder, and agoraphobia in the National Comorbidity Survey Replication. *Archives of General Psychiatry*, 63(4), 415–424.

Khosravani, V., Nikcevic, A.V., Spada, M.M., Samimi Ardestani, S.M. & Najafi, M. (2024). The independent contribution of positive and negative metacognitions about smoking to urge to smoke, withdrawal symptoms and dependence in smoking-dependent men. *Clinical psychology and psychotherapy*, 31(4), e3024.

Killikelly, C. & Maercker, A. (2018). Prolonged grief disorder for ICD-11: The primacy of clinical utility and international applicability. *European Journal of Psychotraumatology*, 8(6), 1476441.

Kim, S.T., Park, C.I., Kim, H.W., Jeon, S., Kang, J.I. & Kim, S.J. (2021). Dysfunctional metacognitive beliefs in patients with obsessive-compulsive disorder and pattern of their changes following a 3-month treatment. *Frontiers in Psychiatry*, 12, 628985.

Knowles, M.M., Foden, P., El-Deredy, W. & Wells, A. (2016). A systematic review of efficacy of the attention training technique in clinical and nonclinical samples. *Journal of Clinical Psychology*, 72(10), 999–1025.

Knowles, M.M. & Wells, A. (2018). Single dose of the attention training technique increases resting alpha and beta-oscillations in frontoparietal brain networks: A randomized controlled comparison. *Frontiers in Psychology*, 9, 1768.

Köcher, L.M., Schneider, K. & Christiansen, H. (2021). Thinking about worry: A systematic review and meta-analysis on the assessment of metacognitions in children and adolescents. *World Journal of Psychiatry*, 11(9), 635–658.

Kolubinski, D.C., Marino, C., Nikcevic, A.V. & Spada, M.M. (2019). A metacognitive model of self-esteem. *Journal of Affective Disorders*, 256, 42–53.

Kolubinski, D.C., Nikcevic, A.V., Lawrence, J.A. & Spada, M.M. (2016). The role of metacognition in self-critical rumination: An investigation in individuals presenting with low self-esteem. *Journal of Rational-Emotive & Cognitive-Behavior Therapy*, 34(1), 73–85.

Koolhaas, J.M., Bartolomucci, A., Buwalda, B., de Boer, S.F., Flügge, G., ... & Fuchs, E. (2011). Stress revisited: A critical evaluation of the stress concept. *Neuroscience and Biobehavioral Reviews*, 35(5), 1291–1301.

Kovács, L.N., Takacs, Z.K., Tóth, Z., Simon, E., Schmelowszky, Á. & Kökönyei, G. (2020). Rumination in major depressive and bipolar disorder: A meta-analysis. *Journal of Affective Disorders*, 276, 1131–1141.

Kroener, J., Eickholt, M.L., & Sosic-Vasic, Z. (2024). Group based metacognitive therapy for alcohol use disorder: A pilot study. *Frontiers of Psychiatry*. June 28:15:1375960.doi:10.3389/fpsyt.2024.1375960.

Kubiak, T., Zahn, D., Siewert, K., Jonas, C. & Weber, H. (2014). Positive beliefs about rumination are associated with ruminative thinking and affect in daily life: Evidence for a metacognitive view on depression. *Behavioural and Cognitive Psychotherapy*, 42(5), 568–576.

Lassemo, E., Sandanger, I., Nygård, J.F. & Sørgaard, K.W. (2017). The epidemiology of post-traumatic stress disorder in Norway: Trauma characteristics and pre-existing psychiatric disorders. *Social Psychiatry and Psychiatric Epidemiology*, 52 (1), 11–19.

Lawson, R., Carter, J.D., Britt, E., Knowles, K., Then, R., ... & Tauamiti, R. (2022). Modified metacognitive therapy for anorexia nervosa: An open trial in an outpatient setting. *The International Journal of Eating Disorders*, 55(7), 983–989.

Leigh-Hunt, N., Bagguley, D., Bash, K., Turner, V., Turnbull, S., ... & Caan, W. (2017). An overview of systematic reviews on the public health consequences of social isolation and loneliness. *Public Health*, 152, 157–171.

Lenzo, V., Sardella, A., Martino, G. & Quattropani, M.C. (2020). A systematic review of metacognitive beliefs in chronic medical conditions. *Frontiers in Psychology*, 10, 2875.

Lievaart, M., Huijding, J., van der Veen, F.M., Hovens, J.E. & Franken, I.H. (2017). The impact of angry rumination on anger-primed cognitive control. *Journal of Behavior Therapy and Experimental Psychiatry*, 54, 135–142.

Limburg, K., Watson, H.J., Hagger, M.S. & Egan, S.J. (2017). The relationship between perfectionism and psychopathology: A meta-analysis. *Journal of Clinical Psychology*, 73(10), 1301–1326.

Maher-Edwards, L., Fernie, B.A., Murphy, G., Nikcevic, A.V. & Spada, M.M. (2012). Metacognitive factors in chronic fatigue syndrome. *Clinical Psychology & Psychotheraphy*, 19(6), 552–557.

Mansueto, G., Caselli, G., Ruggiero, G.M. & Sassaroli, S. (2019). Metacognitive beliefs and childhood adversities: An overview of the literature. *Psychology, Health & Medicine*, 24(5), 542–550.

Mansueto, G., Jarach, A., Caselli, G., Ruggiero, G.M., Sassaroli, S., Nikcevic, A., Spada, M.M. & Palmieri, S. (2024) A systematic review of the relationship between generic and specific metacognitive beliefs and emotion dysregulation. *Clinical Psychology and Psychotherapy*, 31(1), e2961.

Mansueto, G., Martino, F., Palmieri, S., Scaini, S., Ruggiero, G.M., Sassaroli, S. & Caselli, G. (2019). Desire thinking across addictive behaviours: A systematic review and meta-analysis. *Addictive Behaviors*, 98, 106018.

Martino, F., Caselli, G., Di Tommaso, J., Sassaroli, S., Spada, M.M., Valenti, B., Berardi, D., Sasdelli, A. & Menchetti, M. (2018). Anger and depressive ruminations as predictors of dysregulated behaviours in borderline personality disorder. *Clinical Psychology & Psychotherapy*, 25(2), 188–194.

Martino, F., Caselli, G., Felicetti, F., Rampioni, M., Romanelli, P., Troiani, L., Sassaroli, S., Albery, I.P. & Spada, M.M. (2017). Desire thinking as a predictor of craving and binge drinking: A longitudinal study. *Addictive Behaviors*, 64, 118–122.

Martino, F., Caselli, G., Fiabane, E., Felicetti, F., Trevisani, C., Menchetti, M., Mezzaluna, C., Sassaroli, S., Albery, I.P. & Spada, M.M. (2019). Desire thinking as a predictor of drinking status following treatment for alcohol use disorder: A prospective study. *Addictive Behaviors*, 95, 70–76.

McEvoy, P.M., Erceg-Hurn, D.M., Anderson, R.A., Campbell, B.N. & Nathan, P.R. (2015). Mechanisms of change during group metacognitive therapy for repetitive negative thinking in primary and non-primary generalized anxiety disorder. *Journal of Anxiety Disorders*, 35, 19–26.

McLaughlin, K.A., Aldao, A., Wisco, B.E. & Hilt, L.M. (2014). Rumination as a trans- diagnostic factor underlying transitions between internalizing symptoms and aggressive behavior in early adolescents. *Journal of Abnormal Psychology*, 123 (1), 13–23.

McLaughlin, K.A. & Nolen-Hoeksema, S. (2011). Rumination as a transdiagnostic factor in depression and anxiety. *Behaviour Research and Therapy*, 49(3), 186–193.

McPhillips, R., Salmon, P., Wells, A. & Fisher, P. (2019). Qualitative analysis of emotional distress in cardiac patients from the perspectives of cognitive behavioral and metacognitive theories: Why might cognitive behavioral therapy have limited benefit, and might metacognitive therapy be more effective? *Frontiers in Psychology*, 9, 2288.

Melchior, K., van der Heiden, C., Deen, M., Mayer, B. & Franken, I.H.A. (2023). The effectiveness of metacognitive therapy in comparison to exposure and response prevention for obsessive-compulsive disorder: A randomized controlled trial. *Journal of Obsessive-Compulsive and Related Disorders*, 36, 100780.

Meyer, T.J., Miller, M.L., Metzger, R.L. & Borkovec, T.D. (1990). Development and validation of the Penn State Worry Questionnaire. *Behaviour Research and Therapy*, 28, 487–495.

Molina, S. & Borkovec, T.D. (1994). The Penn State Worry Questionnaire: Psychometric properties and associated characteristics. In: G.C.L. Davey & F. Tallis (eds.), *Worrying: Perspectives on theory, assessment and treatment* (pp. 265–283). Wiley.

Moncrieff, J., Cooper, R.E., Stockmann, T., Amendola, S., Hengartner, M.P. & Horowitz, M.A. (2022). The serotonin theory of depression: A systematic umbrella review of the evidence. *Molecular psychiatry*, 28(8), 3243–3256.

Morrison, A.P., Pyle, M., Chapman, N., French, P., Parker, S.K. & Wells, A. (2014). Metacognitive therapy in people with a schizophrenia spectrum diagnosis and medication resistant symptoms: A feasibility study. *Journal of Behavior Therapy and Experimental Psychiatry*, 45(2), 280–284.

Morrison, A.P. & Wells, A. (2007). Relationships between worry, psychotic experiences and emotional distress in patients with schizophrenia spectrum diagnoses and comparisons with anxious and non-patient groups. *Behaviour Research and Therapy*, 45(7), 1593–1600.

Muñoz-Navarro, R., Medrano, L.A., Limonero, J.T., González-Blanch, C., Moriana, J.A., ... & Cano-Vindel, A. (2022). The mediating role of emotion regulation in trans- diagnostic cognitive behavioural therapy for emotional disorders in primary care: Secondary analyses of the PsicAP randomized controlled trial. *Journal of Affective Disorders*, 303, 206–215.

Murray, J., Scott, H., Connolly, C. & Wells, A. (2018). The attention training technique improves children's ability to delay gratification: A controlled comparison with progressive relaxation. *Behaviour Research and Therapy*, 104, 1–6.

Murray, J., Theakston, A. & Wells, A. (2016). Can the attention training technique turn one marshmallow into two? Improving children's ability to delay gratification. *Behaviour Research and Therapy*, 77, 34–39.

Myers, S., Fisher, P. & Wells, A. (2009). Metacognition and cognition as predictors of obsessive-compulsive symptoms: A prospective study. *International. Journal of Cognitive Psychotherapy*, 2, 132–142.

Myers, S. & Wells, A. (2005). Obsessive-compulsive symptoms: The contribution of metacognitions and responsibility. *Journal of Anxiety Disorders*, 189, 806–817.

Myhr, P., Hursti, T., Emanuelsson, K., Löfgren, E. & Hjemdal, O. (2019). Can the attention training technique reduce stress in students? A controlled study of stress appraisals and meta-worry. *Frontiers in Psychology*, 10, 1532.

Nassif, Y. & Wells, A. (2014). Attention training reduces intrusive thoughts cued by a narrative of stressful life events: A controlled study. *Journal of Clinical Psychology*, 70(6), 510–517.

Natalini, E., Fioretti, A., Riedl, D., Moschen, R. & Eibenstein, A. (2020). Tinnitus and metacognitive beliefs: Results of a cross-sectional observational study. *Brain Sciences*, 11(1), 3.

Nelson, T.O. (1996). Consciousness and metacognition. *American Psychologist*, 51 (2), 102–116.

Newman, M.G., Zuellig, A.R., Kachin, K.E., Constantino, M.J., Przeworski, A., ... & Cashman- McGrath, L. (2002). Preliminary reliability and validity of the Generalized Anxiety Disorder Questionnaire-IV: A revised self-report diagnostic measure of generalized anxiety disorder. *Behavior Therapy*, 33(2), 215–233.

Nolen-Hoeksema, S. (1991). Responses to depression and their effects on the duration of depressive episodes. *Journal of Abnormal Psychology*, 100(4), 569–582.

Nolen-Hoeksema, S. (2000). The role of rumination in depressive disorders and mixed anxiety/depressive symptoms. *Journal of Abnormal Psychology*, 109(3), 504–511.

Nolen-Hoeksema, S. & Watkins, E.R. (2011). A heuristic for developing transdiagnostic models of psychopathology: Explaining multifinality and divergent trajectories. *Perspectives on Psychological Science: A Journal of the Association for Psychological Science*, 6(6), 589–609.

Nolen-Hoeksema, S., Wisco, B.E. & Lyubomirsky, S. (2008). Rethinking rumination. *Perspectives on Psychological Science: A Journal of the Association for Psychological Science*, 3(5), 400–424.

Nordahl, H., Anyan, F. & Hjemdal, O. (2023). Prospective relations between dysfunctional metacognitive beliefs, metacognitive strategies, and anxiety: Results from a four-wave longitudinal mediation model. *Behavior Therapy*, 54(5), 765–776.

Nordahl, H., Anyan, F., Hjemdal, O. & Wells, A. (2022). Metacognition, cognition and social anxiety: A test of temporal and reciprocal relationships. *Journal of Anxiety Disorders*, 86, 102516.

Nordahl, H., Hjemdal, O., Hagen, R., Nordahl, H.M. & Wells, A. (2019). What lies beneath trait-anxiety? Testing the self-regulatory executive function model of vulnerability. *Frontiers in Psychology*, 10, 122.

Nordahl, H., Nordahl, H.M., Hjemdal, O. & Wells, A. (2017). Cognitive and metacognitive predictors of symptom improvement following treatment for social anxiety disorder: A secondary analysis from a randomized controlled trial. *Clinical Psychology & Psychotherapy*, 24, 1221–1227.

Nordahl, H., Nordahl, H.M., Vogel, P.A. & Wells, A. (2018). Explaining depression symptoms in patients with social anxiety disorder: Do maladaptive metacognitive beliefs play a role? *Clinical Psychology & Psychotherapy*, 25(3), 457–464.

Nordahl, H. & Wells, A. (2017). Testing the metacognitive model against the benchmark CBT model of social anxiety disorder: Is it time to move beyond cognition? *PLoS One*, 12(5), e0177109.

Nordahl, H.M. (2016). The effectiveness of MCT on anxiety and depression: The Trondheim randomized controlled trials. Presentation at the 3rd International Conference of Metacognitive Therapy, Milan, 8–9 April 2016.

Nordahl, H.M., Borkovec, T.D., Hagen, R., Kennair, L.E.O., Hjemdal, O., ... & Wells, A. (2018). Metacognitive therapy versus cognitive-behavioural therapy in adults with generalised anxiety disorder. *BJ Psych Open*, 4(5), 393–400.

Nordahl, H.M., Vogel, P.A., Morken, G., Stiles, T.C., Sandvik, P. & Wells A. (2016). Paroxetine, cognitive therapy or their combination in the treatment of social anxiety disorder with and without avoidant personality disorder: A randomized clinical trial. *Psychotherapy and Psychosomatics*, 85(6), 346–356.

Nordahl, H.M. & Wells, A. (2019). Metacognitive therapy of early traumatized patients with borderline personality disorder: A phase-II baseline controlled trial. *Frontiers in Psychology*, 10, 1694.

Nordahl, J., Hjemdal, O., Johnson, S.U. & Nordahl, H.M. (2024). Metacognitive therapy versus exposure-based treatments of posttraumatic stress disorder: A preliminary comparative trial in an ordinary clinical practice. *International Journal of Cognitive Therapy*, 17, 685–699.

Normann, N. & Morina, N. (2018). The efficacy of metacognitive therapy: A systematic review and meta-analysis. *Frontiers in Psychology*, 9, 2211.

Olivari, C., Mansueto, G., Marino, C., Candellari, G., Cericola, J., Binnie, J., Spada, M.M. & Caselli, G. (2025). Metacognitive beliefs and desire thinking as potential maintenance factors of compulsive sexual behavior. *Addictive behaviors*, 161, 108214. Advance online publication.

Olstad, S., Solem, S., Hjemdal, O. & Hagen, R. (2015). Metacognition in eating disorders: Comparison of women with eating disorders, self-reported history of eating disorders or psychiatric problems, and healthy controls. *Eating Behaviors*, 16, 17–22.

Osborne, L.M., Voegtline, K., Standeven, L.R., Sundel, B., Pangtey, M., ... & Payne, J.L. (2021). High worry in pregnancy predicts postpartum depression. *Journal of Affective Disorders*, 294, 701–706.

Öst, L.G. (2008). Cognitive behavior therapy for anxiety disorders: 40 years of progress. *Nordic Journal of Psychiatry*, 62(47), 5–10.

Østefjells, T., Lystad, J.U., Berg, A.O., Hagen, R., Loewy, R., ... & Røssberg, J.I. (2017). Metacognitive beliefs mediate the effect of emotional abuse on depressive and psychotic symptoms in severe mental disorders. *Psychological Medicine*, 47 (13), 2323–2333.

Pajak, R., Langhoff, C., Watson, S. & Kamboj, S. (2013). Phenomenology and thematic content of intrusive imagery in bowel and bladder obsession. *Journal of Obsessive-Compulsive and Related Disorders*, 2, 233–240.

Palagini, L., Ong, J.C. & Riemann, D. (2017). The mediating role of sleep-related metacognitive processes in trait and pre-sleep state hyperarousal in insomnia disorder. *Journal of Psychosomatic Research*, 99, 59–65.

Palmer-Cooper, E.C., Woods, C. & Richardson, T. (2023). The relationship between dysfunctional attitudes, maladaptive perfectionism, metacognition and symptoms of mania and depression in bipolar disorder: The role of self-compassion as a mediating factor. *Journal of Affective Disorders*, 341, 265–274.

Palmieri, S., Mansueto, G., Ruggiero, G.M., Caselli, G., Sassaroli, S. & Spada, M. M. (2021a). Metacognitive beliefs across eating disorders and eating behaviours: A systematic review. *Clinical Psychology & Psychotherapy*, 28(5), 1254–1265.

Palmieri, S., Mansueto, G., Scaini, S., Caselli, G., Sapuppo, W., ... & Ruggiero, G. M. (2021b). Repetitive negative thinking and eating disorders: A meta-analysis of the role of worry and rumination. *Journal of Clinical Medicine*, 10(11), 2448.

Papageorgiou, C., Carlile, K., Thorgaard, S., Waring, H., Haslam, J., ... & Wells, A. (2018). Group cognitive-behavior therapy or group metacognitive therapy for obsessive-compulsive disorder? Benchmarking and comparative effectiveness in a routine clinical service. *Frontiers in Psychology*, 9, 2551.

Papageorgiou, C. & Wells, A. (2000). Treatment of recurrent major depression with attention training. *Cognitive and Behavioral Practice*, 7(4),407–413.

Papageorgiou, C. & Wells, A. (2001a). Positive beliefs about depressive rumination: Development and preliminary validation of a self-report scale. *Behavior Therapy*, 32(1), 13–26.

Papageorgiou, C. & Wells, A. (2001b). Metacognitive beliefs about rumination in recurrent major depression. *Cognitive and Behavioral Practice*, 8, 160–164.

Papageorgiou, C. & Wells, A. (eds.) (2004). *Depressive rumination: Nature, theory and treatment*. Wiley.

Papageorgiou, C., Wells, A. & Meina, L.J. (2001). *Development and preliminary validation of the negative beliefs about rumination scale*. Manuscript in preparation.

Parker, S.K., Mulligan, L.D., Milner, P., Bowe, S. & Palmier-Claus, J.E. (2020). Metacognitive therapy for individuals at high risk of developing psychosis: A pilot study. *Frontiers in Psychology*, 10, 2741.

Parment, G. (2023). *MCT-Metakognitiv terapi, – att förstå och effektivt behandla psykologiska problem.* (MCT-Metacognitive therapy, – understanding and effectively treating psychological problems). Studentlitteratur.

Parola, N., Zendjidjian, X.Y., Alessandrini, M., Baumstarck, K., Loundou, A., ... & Boyer, L. (2017). Psychometric properties of the ruminative response scale-short form in a clinical sample of patients with major depressive disorder. *Patient Preference and Adherence*, 11, 929–937.

Pearl, S.B. & Norton, P.J. (2017). Transdiagnostic versus diagnosis specific cognitive behavioural therapies for anxiety: A meta-analysis. *Journal of Anxiety Disorders*, 46, 11–24.

Pedersen, H., Grønnæss, I., Bendixen, M., Hagen, R. & Kennair, L. (2022). Meta-cognitions and brooding predict depressive symptoms in a community adolescent sample. *BMC Psychiatry*, 22(1), 157.

Pedersen, S.G., Anke, A., Friborg, O., Ørbo, M.C., Løkholm, M., Kirkevold, M., Heiberg, G. & Halvorsen, M.B. (2024). Metacognitive beliefs, mood symptoms, and fatigue four years after a stroke: An explorative study. *Plos one*, 19(6), e0305896.

Penney, A.M., Rachor, G.S. & Deleurme, K.A. (2020). Differentiating the roles of intolerance of uncertainty and negative beliefs about worry across emotional disorders. *Journal of Experimental Psychopathology*, 11(4).

Petrošanec, M., Brekalo, M. & Nakic Radoš, S. (2022). The metacognitive model of rumination and depression in postpartum women. *Psychology and Psychotherapy*, 95(3), 838–852.

Rachman, S. (1977). The conditioning theory of fear-acquisition: A critical examination. *Behaviour Research Therapy*, 15(5), 375–387.

Raes, F. & Hermans, D. (2008). On the mediating role of subtypes of rumination in the relationship between childhood emotional abuse and depressed mood: Brooding versus reflection. *Depression and Anxiety*, 25, 1067–1070.

Rauwenhoff, J.C.C., Hagen, R., Karaliute, M., Hjemdal, O., Kennair, L.E.O., Solem, S., Asarnow, R.F., Einarsen, C., Halvorsen, J.Ø., Paoli, S., Saksvik, S.B., Smevik, H., Storvig, G., Wells, A., Skandsen, T. & Olsen, A. (2024). Metacognitive therapy for people experiencing persistent post-concussion symptoms following mild traumatic brain injury: A preliminary multiple case-series study. *Neurotrauma reports*, 5(1), 890–902.

Reinholdt-Dunne, M.L., Seeberg, I., Blicher, A., Normann, N., Vinberg, M., ... & Miskowiak, K. (2021). Residual anxiety in patients with bipolar disorder in full or partial remission: Metacognitive beliefs and neurocognitive function. *Cognitive Therapy and Research*, 45(1), 179–189.

Reinholdt-Dunne, M.L., Tolstrup, M., Svenstrup, K., Hjemdal, O. & Nordahl, H. (2024). Group metacognitive therapy for pediatric obsessive-compulsive disorder: A pilot study. *Journal of Obsessive-Compulsive and Related Disorders*.

Richman Czégel, M.J., Unoka, Z., Dudas, R.B. & Demetrovics, Z. (2022). Rumination in borderline personality disorder: A meta-analytic review. *Journal of Personality Disorders*, 36(4), 399–412.

Robertson, S. & Strodl, E. (2020). Metacognitive therapy for binge eating disorder: A case series study. *Clinical Psychologist*, 24(2), 143–154.

Rogers, M.L., Gallyer, A.J. & Joiner, T.E. (2021). The relationship between suicide-specific rumination and suicidal intent above and beyond suicidal ideation and other suicide risk factors: A multilevel modeling approach. *Journal of Psychiatric Research*, 137, 506–513.

Rogers, M.L., Gorday, J.Y. & Joiner, T.E. (2021). Examination of characteristics of ruminative thinking as unique predictors of suicide-related outcomes. *Journal of Psychiatric Research*, 139, 1–7.

Rogers, M.L. & Joiner, T.E. (2018). Suicide-specific rumination relates to lifetime suicide attempts above and beyond a variety of other suicide risk factors. *Journal of Psychiatric Research*, 98, 78–86.

Rück, C. (2020). *Olyckliga i paradiset: Varför mår vi så dåligt när allt är så bra?* [Unhappy in the paradise: Why do we feel so bad when everything is so good?] Natur & Kultur.

Rusting, C.L. & Nolen-Hoeksema, S. (1998). Regulating responses to anger: Effects of rumination and distraction on angry mood. *Journal of Personality and Social Psychology*, 74(3), 790–803.

Salguero, J.M., García-Sancho, E., Ramos-Cejudo, J. & Kannis-Dymand, L. (2020). Individual differences in anger and displaced aggression: The role of metacognitive beliefs and anger rumination. *Aggressive Behavior*, 46(2), 162–169.

Salkovskis, P.M. (1985). Obsessional-compulsive problems: A cognitive-behavioural analysis. *Behaviour Research and Therapy*, 23(5), 571–583.

Sassaroli, S., Centorame, F., Caselli, G., Favaretto, E., Fiore, F., ... & Rapee, R.M. (2015). Anxiety control and metacognitive beliefs mediate the relationship between inflated responsibility and obsessive compulsive symptoms. *Psychiatry Research*, 228(3), 560–564.

Sauer-Zavala, S., Gutner, C.A., Farchione, T.J., Boettcher, H.T., Bullis, J.R. & Barlow, D.H. (2017). Current definitions of "transdiagnostic" in treatment development: A search for consensus. *Behavior Therapy*, 48(1), 128–138.

SBU (2010). *Behandling av sömnbesvär hos vuxna. En systematisk litteraturöversikt.* [Treatment of sleep problems among adults. A systematic literature review]. SBU-rapport nr 199. Statens beredning för medicinsk och social utvärdering. [SBU report no. 199. Swedish agency for health technology assessment and assessment of social services].

SBU (2020). Fakta om posttraumatisk stress PTSD. [Facts on posttraumatic stress PTSD]. Statens beredning för medicinsk och social utvärdering. [Swedish agency for health technology assessment and assessment of social services].

Schacter, D.L., Chiu, C.Y. & Ochsner, K.N. (1993). Implicit memory: A selective review. *Annual Review of Neuroscience*, 16, 159–182.

Schaich, A., Outzen, J., Assmann, N., Gebauer, C., Jauch-Chara, K., Alvarez-Fischer, D., Hüppe, M., Wells, A., Schweiger, U., Klein, J.P. & Fassbinder, E. (2023). The effectiveness of metacognitive therapy compared to behavioral activation for severely depressed outpatients: A single-center randomized trial. *Psychotherapy and Psychosomatics*, 92(1), 38–48.

Schmidt, R.E., Harvey, A.G. & Van der Linden, M. (2011). Cognitive and affective control in insomnia. *Frontiers in Psychology*, 2, 349.

Schultz, K., Kannis-Dymand, L., Jamieson, D., McLoughlin, L.T., Loughnan, S., Allen, A. & Hermens, D.F. (2023). Examining the longitudinal relationship between metacognitive beliefs and psychological distress in an adolescent population: A preliminary analysis. *Child Psychiatry & Human development*. 1–11.

Schütze, R., Rees, C., Slater, H., Smith, A. & O'Sullivan, P. (2017). "I call it stinkin' thinkin'": A qualitative analysis of metacognition in people with chronic low back pain and elevated catastrophizing. *British Journal of Health Psychology*, 22(3), 463–480.

Schütze, R., Rees, C., Smith, A., Slater, H. & O'Sullivan P. (2020). Metacognition, perseve- rative thinking, and pain catastrophizing: A moderated-mediation analysis. *European Journal of Pain*, 24(1), 223–233.

Selby, E.A., Anestis, M.D. & Joiner, T.E. (2008). Understanding the relationship between emotional and behavioral dysregulation: Emotional cascades. *Behaviour Research and Therapy*, 46(5), 593–611.

Selby, E.A., Kranzler, A., Panza, E. & Fehling, K.B. (2016). Bidirectional-compounding rumination. *Journal of Personality*, 84, 139–153.

Sella, E., Cellini, N., Miola, L., Sarlo, M. & Borella, E. (2019). The influence of metacognitive beliefs on sleeping difficulties in older adults. *Applied Psychology: Health and Well-Being*, 11(1), 20–41.

Sellers, R., Gaweda, Ł., Wells, A. & Morrison, A.P. (2016). The role of unhelpful meta- cognitive beliefs in psychosis: Relationships with positive symptoms and negative affect. *Psychiatry Research*, 246, 401–406.

Sellers, R., Varese, F., Wells, A. & Morrison, A.P. (2017). A meta-analysis of meta-cognitive beliefs as implicated in the self-regulatory executive function model in clinical psychosis. *Schizophrenia Research*, 179, 75–84.

Shafran, R., Booth, R. & Rachman, S. (1993). The reduction of claustrophobia II: Cognitive analyses. *Behaviour Research and Therapy*, 31(1), 75–85.

Simons, M. & Vloet, T.D. (2018). Emetophobia: A metacognitive therapeutic approach for an overlooked disorder. *Z Kinder Jugendpsychiatr Psychother*, 46(1), 57–66.

Skinner, B.F. (1974). *About behaviorism*. Knopf.

Smith, K.E., Mason, T.B., Anderson, N.L. & Lavender, J.M. (2019). Unpacking cognitive emotion regulation in eating disorder psychopathology: The differential relationships between rumination, thought suppression, and eating disorder symptoms among men and women. *Eating Behaviors*, 32, 95–100.

Smith, K.E., Mason, T.B. & Lavender, J.M. (2018). Rumination and eating disorder psycho- pathology: A meta-analysis. *Clinical Psychology Review*, 61, 9–23.

Socialstyrelsen (2003). *Utmattningssyndrom: stressrelaterad psykisk ohälsa* [Exhaustion syndrome: stress related mental illness]. Socialstyrelsen [National Board of Social Affairs and Health].

Socialstyrelsen (2019). *Vård vid depression och ångestsyndrom 2019*. Underlagsrapport. [Care at depression and anxiety syndromes 2019. Background report]. Artikel nummer 2019–2015-13. Socialstyrelsen [National Board of Social Affairs and Health].

Socialstyrelsen (2021). *Nationella riktlinjer för vård av depression och ångestsyndrom* [National guidelines for care/treatment of depression and anxiety syndromes]. Socialstyrelsen [National Board of Social Affairs and Health].

Solem, S., Hagen, R., Hoksnes, J.J. & Hjemdal, O. (2016). The metacognitive model of depression: An empirical test in a large Norwegian sample. *Psychiatry Research*, 242, 171–173.

Solem, S., Haland, A.T., Vogel, P.A., Hansen, B. & Wells, A. (2009). Change in meta- cognitions predicts outcome in obsessive-compulsive disorder patients undergoing treatment with exposure and response prevention. *Behaviour Research and Therapy*, 47, 301–307.

Solem, S., Kennair, L.E.O., Hagen, R., Havnen, A., Nordahl, H.M., ... & Hjemdal, O. (2019). Metacognitive therapy for depression: A 3-year follow-up study assessing recovery, relapse, work force participation, and quality of life. *Frontiers in Psychology*, 10, 2908.

Solem, S., Wells, A., Kennair, L.E.O., Hagen, R., Nordahl, H. & Hjemdal, O. (2021). Metacognitive therapy versus cognitive–behavioral therapy in adults with generalized anxiety disorder: A 9-year follow-up study. *Brain and Behavior*, 11(10), 1–7.

Spada, M.M., Caselli, G., Nikcevic, A.V. & Wells A. (2015). Metacognition in addictive behaviors. *Addictive Behaviors*, 44, 9–15.

Spada, M.M., Caselli, G. & Wells, A. (2013). A triphasic metacognitive formulation of problem drinking. *Clinical Psychology & Psychotherapy*, 20(6), 494–500.

Spada, M.M., Challoner, H., Nikcevic, A., Fernie, B. & Caselli, G. (2016). Metacognitive beliefs about worry and pain catastrophizing as mediators between neuroticism and pain behaviour. *Clinical Psychologist*, 20, 138–146.

Spada, M.M., Moneta, G.B. & Wells, A. (2007). The relative contribution of metacognitive beliefs and alcohol expectancies to drinking behaviour. *Alcohol and Alcoholism*, 42, 567–574.

Spada, M.M., Nikcevic, A.V., Kolubinski, D.C., Offredi, A., Giuri, S., ... & Caselli, G. (2021). Metacognitions, rumination, and worry in personality disorder. *Journal of Affective Disorders*, 293, 117–123.

Spada, M.M., Nikcevic, A.V., Moneta, G.B. & Wells, A. (2008). Metacognition, perceived stress, and negative emotion. *Personality and Individual Differences*, 44(5), 1172–1181.

Spendelow, J.S., Simonds, L.M. & Avery, R.E. (2017). The relationship between co-rumination and internalizing problems: A systematic review and meta-analysis. *Clinical Psychology & Psychotherapy*, 24(2), 512–527.

Startup, H.M. & Erickson, T.M. (2006). The Penn State Worry Questionnaire (PSWQ). In: G.C.L. Davey & A. Wells (eds.), *Worry and its psychological disorders: Theory, assessment and treatment* (pp. 101–119). Wiley.

Startup, H., Pugh, K., Dunn, G., Cordwell, J., Mander, H., ... & Freeman, D. (2016). Worry processes in patients with persecutory delusions. *The British Journal of Clinical Psychology*, 55(4), 387–400.

Staugaard, S.R. (2010). Threatening faces and social anxiety: A literature review. *Clinical Psychology Review*, 30, 669–690.

Strand, E.R., Anyan, F., Hjemdal, O., Nordahl, H.M. & Nordahl, H. (2024). Dysfunctional attitudes versus metacognitive beliefs as within-person predictors of depressive symptoms over time. *Behavior Therapy*, 55(4), 801–812.

Strand, E.R., Hagen, R., Hjemdal, O., Kennair, L.E.O. & Solem, S. (2018). Metacognitive therapy for depression reduces interpersonal problems: Results from a randomized controlled trial. *Frontiers in Psychology*, 9, 1415.

Strand, E.R. & Nordahl, H. (2024). Do patients' interpersonal problems improve following metacognitive therapy? A systematic review and meta-analysis. *Clinical Psychology & Psychotherapy*, 31(2), e2973.

Sun, X., So, S.H., Chan, R., Chiu, C.D. & Leung, P. (2019). Worry and metacognitions as predictors of the development of anxiety and paranoia. *Scientific Reports*, 9(1), 14723.

Sun, X., Zhu, C. & So, S.H.W. (2017). Dysfunctional metacognition across psychopathologies: A meta-analytic review. *European Psychiatry*, 45, 139–153.

Sveriges Psykologförbund (1998). *Yrkesetiska principer för psykologer i Norden antagna av Sveriges psykologförbunds kongress 1998*. Sveriges psykologförbund. [Professional ethics for psychologists in the Nordic countries adopted by the congress in 1998. Swedish psychological association].

Takano, K., Iijima, Y. & Tanno, Y. (2012). Repetitive thought and self-reported sleep disturbance. *Behavior Therapy*, 43(4), 779–789.

Taylor-Bennett, J., Capobianco, L., Wisely, J. & Wells, A. (2024). Qualitative analysis of emotional distress in burns, plastic and reconstructive surgery patients from the perspectives of cognitive and metacognitive models. *Frontiers in Psychiatry*, 15, 1461387.

Techmann, B.A., Joormann, J., Steinman, S.A. & Gotlib, I.H. (2010). Automaticity in anxiety disorders and major depressive disorder. *Clinical Psychology Review*, 32, 575–603.

Tenti, M., Raffaeli, W., Fontemaggi, A. & Gremigni, P. (2023). The relationship between metacognition, anger, and pain intensity among fibromyalgia patients: A serial mediation model. *Psychology, Health & Medicine*, 29(4), 791–808.

Thielsch, C., Andor, T. & Ehring, T. (2015). Do metacognitions and intolerance of uncertainty predict worry in everyday life? An ecological momentary assessment study. *Behavior Therapy*, 46(4), 532–543.

Thingbak, A., Capobianco, L., Wells, A. & O'Toole, M.S. (2024). Relationships between metacognitive beliefs and anxiety and depression in children and adolescents: A meta-analysis. *Journal of Affective Disorders* 361, (15) 36–50.

Törneke, N. (2010). *Learning RFT: An introduction to relational frame theory and its clinical application.* Context Press/New Harbinger Publications.

Törneke, N. (2014). *Relationsinramningsteori – RFT: Teori och klinisk tillämpning* [Relational frame theory – RFT: Theory and clinical applications]. Studentlitteratur.

Treynor, W., Gonzalez, R. & Nolen-Hoeksema, S. (2003). Rumination reconsidered: A psychometric analysis. *Cognitive Therapy and Research*, 27(3), 247–259.

Trick, L., Watkins, E., Windeatt, S. & Dickens, C. (2016). The association of perseverative negative thinking with depression, anxiety and emotional distress in people with long term conditions: A systematic review. *Journal of Psychosomatic Research*, 91, 89–101.

van der Heiden, C. & Melchior, K. (2014). A 30-month follow-up of generalized anxiety disorder: Status after metacognitive therapy and intolerance of uncertainty-therapy. *European Journal for Person Centered Healthcare*, 2, 434–438.

van der Heiden, C., Muris, P. & van der Molen, H.T. (2012). Randomized controlled trial on the effectiveness of metacognitive therapy and intolerance-of-uncertainty therapy for generalized anxiety disorder. *Behaviour Research and Therapy*, 50(2), 100–109.

van der Heiden, C.V., Rossen, K.V., Dekker, A., Damstra, M.F. & Deen, M.L. (2016). Metacognitive therapy for obsessive–compulsive disorder: A pilot study. *Journal of Obsessive-Compulsive and Related Disorders*, 9, 24–29.

Wang, S., Jing, H., Chen, L. & Li, Y. (2020). The influence of negative life events on suicidal ideation in college students: The role of rumination. *International Journal of Environmental Research and Public Health*, 17(8), 2646.

Wells, A. (1994). A multi-dimensional measure of worry: Development and preliminary validation of the Anxious Thoughts Inventory. *Anxiety, Stress and Coping: An International Journal*, 6, 289–299.

Wells, A. (1995). Meta-cognition and worry: A cognitive model of generalised anxiety disorder. *Behavioral and Cognitive Psychotherapy*, 23, 301–320.

Wells, A. (1997). *Cognitive therapy of anxiety disorders: A practice manual and conceptual guide.* Wiley.

Wells, A. (2000). *Emotional disorders and metacognition: Innovative cognitive therapy.* Wiley.

Wells, A. (2005a). The metacognitive model of GAD: Assessment of meta-worry and relationship with DSM-IV generalized anxiety disorder. *Cognitive Therapy and Research*, 29, 107–121.

Wells, A. (2005b). Detached mindfulness in cognitive therapy: A metacognitive analysis and ten techniques. *Journal of Rational-Emotive & Cognitive-Behavior Therapy*, 23(4), 337–355.

Wells, A. (2009). *Metacognitive therapy for anxiety and depression.* Guilford.

Wells, A. (2010). Metacognitive theory and therapy for worry and generalized anxiety disorder: Review and status. *Journal of Experimental Psychopathology*, 1(1), 133–145.

Wells A. (2019). Breaking the cybernetic code: Understanding and treating the human metacognitive control system to enhance mental health. *Frontiers in Psychology*, 10, 2621.

Wells, A., Capobianco, L., Matthews, G. & Nordahl, H.M. (2020). Editorial: Metacognitive therapy: Science and practice of a paradigm. *Frontiers in Psychology*, 11, 576210.

Wells, A. & Cartwright-Hatton, S. (2004). A short form of the Metacognitions Questionnaire: Properties of the MCQ-30. *Behaviour Research and Therapy*, 42 (4), 385–396.

Wells, A. & Davies, M. (1994). The Thought Control Questionnaire: A measure of individual differences in control of unwanted thoughts. *Behaviour Research and Therapy*, 32, 871–878.

Wells, A. & Faija, C. (2018). Metacognitive therapy for anxiety and depression in cardiac rehabilitation: Commentary on the UK National Institute of Health Research funded PATHWAY programme. *Journal of Cardiology and Cardiovascular Sciences*, 2, 10–14.

Wells, A., Gwilliam, P. & Cartwright-Hatton, S. (2001). The thought fusion instrument. Unpublished self-report scale. University of Manchester.

Wells, A. & Matthews, G. (1994). *Attention and emotion: A clinical perspective.* Erlbaum.

Wells, A. & Matthews, G. (1996). Modelling cognition in emotional disorder: The S-REF model. *Behaviour Research and Therapy*, 34, 881–888.

Wells, A. & Papageorgiou, C. (1998). Relationships between worry, obsessive-compulsive symptoms and meta-cognitive beliefs. *Behaviour Research and Therapy*, 36 (9), 899–913.

Wells, A., Reeves, D., Capobianco, L., Heal, C., Davies, L., … & Fisher, P. (2021). Improving the effectiveness of psychological interventions for depression and anxiety in cardiac rehabilitation: PATHWAY – a single-blind, parallel, randomized, controlled trial of group metacognitive therapy. *Circulation*, 144(1), 23–33.

Wells, A., Reeves, D., Heal, C., Davies, L.M., Shields, G.E., … & Capobianco, L. (2022a). Evaluating metacognitive therapy to improve treatment of anxiety and depression in cardiovascular disease: The NIHR funded PATHWAY research programme. *Frontiers in Psychiatry*, 13, 886407.

Wells, A., Reeves, D., Heal, C., Fisher, P., Doherty, P., … & Capobianco, L. (2022b). Metacognitive therapy self-help for anxiety-depression: Single-blind randomized feasibility trial in cardiovascular disease. *Health Psychology: Official Journal of the Division of Health Psychology, American Psychological Association*, 41(5), 366–377.

Wells, A., Reeves, D., Heal, C., Fisher, P., Doherty, P., … & Capobianco, L. (2023). Metacognitive therapy home-based self-help for anxiety and depression in cardiovascular disease patients in the UK: A single-blind randomised controlled trial. *PLoS Medicine*, 20(1), e1004161.

Wells, A., Walton, D., Lovell, K. & Proctor, D. (2015). Metacognitive therapy versus prolonged exposure in adults with chronic post-traumatic stress disorder: A parallel randomized controlled trial. *Cognitive Therapy and Research*, 39, 70–80.

Wells, A., Welford, M., King, P., Papageorgiou, C., Wisely, J. & Mendel, E. (2010). A pilot randomized trial of metacognitive therapy vs applied relaxation in the treatment of adults with generalized anxiety disorder. *Behaviour Research and Therapy*, 48(5), 429–434.

Wenn, J., O'Connor, M., Breen, L.J. & Rees, C.S. (2019b). Exploratory study of metacognitive beliefs about coping processes in prolonged grief symptomatology. *Death Studies*, 43(3), 143–153.

Wenn, J.A., O'Connor, M., Kane, R.T., Rees, C.S. & Breen, L.J. (2019a). A pilot randomised controlled trial of metacognitive therapy for prolonged grief. *BMJ Open*, 9(1), e021409.

Wilhelm, F.H. & Roth, W.T. (1997). Clinical characteristics of flight phobia. *Journal of Anxiety Disorders*, 11(3), 241–261.

Wilkinson, P.O., Croudace, T.J. & Goodyer, I.M. (2013). Rumination, anxiety, depressive symptoms and subsequent depression in adolescents at risk for psychopathology: A longitudinal cohort study. *BMC Psychiatry*, 13, 250.

Winter, L., Schweiger, U. & Kahl, K.G. (2020). Feasibility and outcome of metacognitive therapy for major depressive disorder: A pilot study. *BMC Psychiatry*, 20, 566.

Young, J.E. & Beck, A.T. (1980). Cognitive therapy scale. Unpublished manuscript, University of Pennsylvania.

Young, J.E., Klosko, J.S. & Weismaar, M.E. (2006). *Schema therapy: A practitioner's guide*. Guilford.

Ziadni, M.S., Sturgeon, J.A. & Darnall, B.D. (2018). The relationship between negative metacognitive thoughts, pain catastrophizing and adjustment to chronic pain. *European Journal of Pain*, 22(4), 756–762.

Index

For Product Safety Concerns and Information please contact our EU
representative GPSR@taylorandfrancis.com
Taylor & Francis Verlag GmbH, Kaufingerstraße 24, 80331 München, Germany